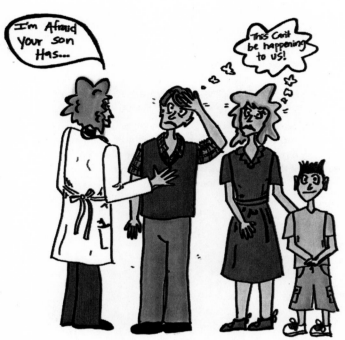

PARENTS
of Children with Disabilities

A SURVIVAL GUIDE
FOR FATHERS & MOTHERS

LIBERTY
UNIVERSITY
BOOKS

Parents of Children with Disabilities
by Press Barnhill, D.B.A. & Gena P. Barnhill, Ph.D.

ISBN-13: 978-0-9819357-8-2

Cover & Interior Design:

Megan Johnson
Johnson2Design
Johnson2Design.com

Illustrations:

Salem Hicks

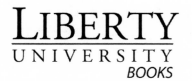

A Division of Liberty University Press
Lynchburg, VA

This book is dedicated to parents of all ages
who have been given the opportunity to love
and support a child with a disability.

To

GRADYS

Blessings.

Press

ACKNOWLEDGEMENTS

We first want to thank the hundreds of parents that we had the opportunity to meet and share our lives with in our support group. Thank you for opening up yourselves to us and to fellow parents and for caring enough to ask for help. We certainly want to thank the three families that shared their personal stories. Thank you Susan, Carl, and Tyler and Becky as your stories are truly inspirational to all of us. We also need to thank our son Brent for allowing us to discuss his story and share how he has had such an important impact on our family. This book could not have been written without him.

Except for our story and the three family stories, all other stories were created by the authors. The characters and situations are not based on any specific person or persons, but rather are a synthesis of stories we have heard or known about in our work with families.

TABLE OF CONTENTS

PREFACE

O ur country has a long history of hero worship. We focus much of our energies on outstanding athletes, powerful politicians, technological geniuses, business magnates, religious leaders, media darlings, and many others occupying niches of broad or narrow scope. However, we also have the wisdom, oftentimes, to understand that heroes are not really those that are cast in the limelight, appearing in the newspaper or on television regularly, or being well-rewarded financially for whatever special trait they seem to exhibit. Rather, we increasingly realize that we find heroes in persons who simply make a great impact on their families, their friends, their communities, and ultimately, in their own way, on the world.

For the last 40 years, my professional affiliation has been in the world of disabilities. As a special educator, I have been fortunate to observe the work of many heroes. Most of these persons—teachers, administrators, and parents – have received little recognition beyond the scope of their schools, homes, and immediate communities. But I have learned that this is where differences are made, where lives are made special, and where futures are made more positive.

Press and Gena Barnhill are heroes. They are heroes because of their lives and their commitment to their family and to others. They are no doubt embarrassed to be referred to as such. They are parents who are others-centered, hang in there, learn as much as they can, and do whatever they can. They offer us, in this book, an opportunity to appreciate the special challenges, the special opportunities, and the special ways in which parents can respond to having a child with a disability.

I had the good fortune to meet Gena Barnhill for the first time six years ago. Lynchburg College was initiating a program to train teachers to work with students with autism spectrum disorders. Gena came to Lynchburg College for a summer to teach a class, returned to do the same again, and then joined our faculty. I knew that we would have a program of tremendous quality with a professional of her special talents. But I realized later how the experiences that she and Press had had, combined with this professional expertise and their ability to communicate with others, would have such a profound impact on our community, our state, and even internationally as parents and teachers were able to learn so much more about individuals with autism spectrum disorders in particular and individuals with disabilities in general.

This book is a treasure for all that will read it. For parents in general, it will reinforce your efforts as you serve in the most important role that any of us can play in life. For parents of children with disabilities, it will provide you with the sage advice and wisdom of persons who have been there and have experienced the challenges that many face. For teachers and other professionals, it will provide a much broader view on parental perspectives that must be part of your responsibilities within your respective professions.

Press and Gena clearly place their perspectives in a strong foundation of faith. The book seamlessly blends experiences that come from day-to-day life, professional knowledge, and their strong belief in the role of God in their lives. Further, they include selected chapters from friends and colleagues who also offer their unique perspectives based on their experiences with their own child with a disability.

What have I learned from reading this book? More than this preface will hold, but certainly: the special challenges faced by fathers that are too often not central to the discussion of family considerations; the critical nature of keeping families intact in support of each other and their children; the importance of

Parents of Children with Disabilities

friendship from others and mutual support; the reality that healing often occurs in very important ways even in the absence of a prayed-for disability cure; that parental reactions to the knowledge that their child has a disability and to the daily realities and challenges do not lend themselves to a strictly linear model but rather reflect cyclical and unexpected turns; that fairness is a most difficult concept such as when it comes to discipline; the importance of faith for persons with disabilities and their families; and the ways in which all of us can help each other, whether it concerns raising children with disabilities or the myriad of other challenges we all face in life. You will be a better person for having chosen to read this book.

Ed Polloway

Professor of Special Education and

Dean of Graduate Studies at Lynchburg College

INTRODUCTION

G ena met numerous families who had children with disabilities when she worked as a school psychologist in a large school district in Missouri. Frequently these parents described feelings of isolation and confusion as to where to turn for help outside of the school district. We also had experienced intense feelings of isolation and, at times, despair years earlier in our journey parenting our son who has a disability. We became determined that no one should need to feel isolated when raising a child or children with disabilities, regardless of their child's age. We approached our church to request the use of a room to be used to start a support group for families dealing with autism spectrum disorders. The church reluctantly agreed to provide a small room and we scheduled our first meeting for a Monday night in January of 2001. Many parents arrived just before the scheduled starting time, so we needed to move to a larger room. Still more parents showed up several minutes later and we moved again down the hall to an even bigger room. We ended up with about 60 parents in attendance that first night and our parent support group was launched.

One of the things we realized after the first year was that we had a number of good resources to draw upon that parents could use to access help for their children, but no resources to help the parents themselves deal with their very challenging situation. Gena was an expert in autism spectrum disorders and special education disabilities and led quite a few of the meetings talking about topics such as teaching children social skills, individual education plans, services schools could provide, etc. We also had many experts from other support organizations present information to our group. We were able to provide the requested information on educational services, but we began to realize that there were even bigger needs. The parents needed support to help cope with the extra demands on their life as a result of their child's disability. Our support group had grown even larger and we were unable to provide individual support to each parent.

We then began to search for materials to help the parents cope with their personal issues but could find almost nothing. I put together a few programs for fathers and Gena presented some programs to help the mothers. Gradually the idea of writing a book for parents took form. We talked to a few parents and received enthusiastic support for the idea. Press approached Carl about writing his story and he readily agreed. You will find his inspirational story in chapter 11 in the book.

We approached a couple that was parenting their daughter who had severe disabilities from a traumatic birth and Susan's moving and encouraging story is included in our book in chapter 6. A third couple we met, Tyler and Becky agreed to write their story for our book also. Their son suffered a sudden and almost fatal brain hemorrhage at age 12. The difficulties they went through, and the impact on their marriage and their daughters, and the wonderful ways God has blessed them are presented in chapter 13.

The purpose of our book is to provide some insight and inspiration to parents that have a child or children with a disability. This is certainly not a comprehensive effort to cover all the issues, but we selected topics that we found our support group parents really needed help with. This book is NOT another parenting book. There are plenty of good books available on how to parent. This book is specifically written to help the parents themselves deal with their unique situation.

We begin this book, primarily written by Press and from his perspective, with the issues surrounding the early days and months after the child's accident or diagnosis of a disability. This is a critical period that almost everyone is unprepared for. Next we try to provide different perspectives from the point of view of the father and the mother. The next chapters on friendships, discipline, how to help yourself, and mister fix-it address specific issues that many parents struggle with. The chapter on love, circumstances and growth provides some thoughts on how to grow as a person in your relationships. The last two chapters challenge parents to address how they can look at their circumstances from a different perspective and perhaps be inspired to do God's will given their difficult and demanding situation.

We hope and pray that each parent that reads our book will come away with at least a few new ideas, a changed perspective and real hope for the future. We pray that God will bless each and every parent and that you would pass this book on to others who may need encouragement and support in their special journey.

Press and Gena Barnhill

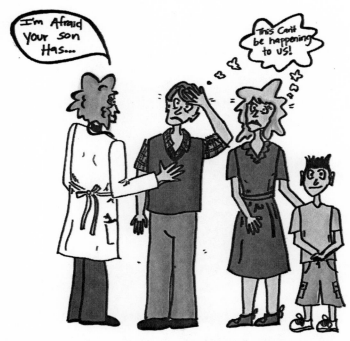

CHAPTER 1
Dashed Expectations

5

P arenting did not turn out as you thought it would. You are the parent of a special child. For most of us, we made this discovery either at birth or in the first few years of our child's life. It could be later as the result of an illness or accident. Most of us can remember when we were told, how we were told, and who told us—and we can remember that sick feeling.

Our first child, Brent, had significant trauma at birth but was apparently fine a few hours later. He was "normal" (at least we thought he was) for the first 4 years. He started having problems relating to the other children in nursery school, and the teacher brought this to our attention. My wife, Gena, was upset and concerned, but I had the usual reaction of what I now call the "Big D"—denial. I remember telling her not to worry; he was just a little immature and would grow out of it. This continued for the next few years until first grade, when it became clear he was continuing to have trouble. We had tests done, we went to therapy, we had many school meetings, and we got lots of different diagnoses.

What Brent really had was Asperger Syndrome, a pervasive developmental disability that many researchers liken to high functioning autism. A correct diagnosis was not made until Brent was 21. It was only after Gena was working on her PhD in behavior disorders and autism that Brent was correctly diagnosed. Asperger Syndrome was not recognized as a formal disorder by the American Psychiatric Association until 1994, and through all of Brent's schooling he had the wrong diagnosis. As a result, the treatment plans were frequently ineffective and discouraging for all concerned.

The impact on our family was at times devastating to me, to Gena, and to our second child, Kristen, who was born a little less than three years after Brent. Brent was placed in special education classes from first grade until the end of eighth grade. His behavior was a constant problem for teachers and administrators, leading to numerous calls to Gena at home. This also led to many meetings with the special education staff and his teachers. These phone calls and meetings were always upsetting and sometimes led to conflicts between Gena and myself on what to do and how to respond. I would frequently deny that the problems were as severe as we were being told, but Gena could see that there were significant problems and they were not going away with time.

After a lot of pushing, Gena finally got all of us to go to family counseling. Kristen and I were very unsupportive and wanted to avoid talking about the problems. Kristen was especially embarrassed about her older brother's behavior and did all she could to separate herself from him. Luckily, they were generally not in the same schools at the same time. I did not want to admit my family was dysfunctional and found this to be embarrassing.

Through most of Brent's first 10 years of school I was denying a long-term problem existed, and I insisted that he would grow out of it. This seemed to be true for a while, as Brent's best two years were his last years of high school. He actually was inducted into the National Honor Society and went off to college the next year. Unfortunately, without the structure of high school, he was unable to handle college and had to return home. This forced me to accept that he was not going to grow out of the problem, and shortly after that Gena started her doctoral courses and was able to identify the correct diagnosis for Brent. Brent is now 33, and there is no denying that his disability is permanent and he needs our help and support for the rest of our lives.

Anger, Blame, and Denial

So, how do most of us first react to such a situation? Many fathers and mothers will get angry—really angry. We get angry about the professionals telling us what

> "What really upsets us is that things will not be as we hoped."

we do not want to hear. We will likely become frustrated and scared. What really upsets us is that things will not be as we hoped. Our child may not be able to participate in sports or play an instrument or even socialize well with other kids. We like to "fix" things and have the answers, but this situation frequently produces more questions than answers. What is this going to cost in time and money and energy? What will be the impact on the marriage, the family, and our careers? What will other people think? It was almost 30 years ago that the nursery teacher first talked to us about her concerns regarding Brent's social skills. I am still dealing with anger due to frustrations and my inability to "fix" the situation.

Lots of questions and, at least initially, there are no obvious answers. One thing many fathers know for sure is that when we get really mad, we need to find someone to blame. The obvious first targets are the doctors, but that wears off after a while. Shooting the messenger rarely does much good. We can blame the child, but the child did not choose to be disabled, so that is really not very fair. We can blame our wife. After all, she brought the child into the world, she is right there, and she is not handling things really well now. Easy target. Again not fair, but you feel you have to blame someone, right?

How about blaming God? Surveys show us that over 90% of North Americans believe in God. He is all powerful, all knowing, and He allowed this to happen. This is especially tough for Christians as we believe that God is in charge, God loves all of us, and yet He allows this innocent person to be disabled! What good does this do? Our perspective is too limited to understand, especially right after we have just received the diagnosis. This situation frequently forces us to either trust God or to blame God. Suffice it to say that I would not be writing this book and Gena would not have her career as an autism educator, and we would not have been facilitating a support group for families dealing with autism spectrum disorders if not for Brent's disability and allowing God to work through us.

Our blaming someone at least gives us somewhere to focus our anger. A lot of parents (especially fathers) stay angry for a long time and unfortunately misdirect their anger to those closest to them such as the spouse, the child, friends, co-workers, even themselves. Clearly this can be very destructive and can lead to the other big D's—depression and divorce. We cover these topics in detail later in the book.

Unfortunately, many parents that have a child with special needs are now single. Frequently, the increased pressure of the child with a disability can become the problem that is too big for the marriage to handle. In our support group, many of the parents were single and the vast majority of these single parents were mothers. Less than 1 in 8 people attending our meetings were fathers.

Is there anything good that comes out of our anger? It all depends on whether we can use our anger to energize ourselves to help the child, the family, and ourselves, or not. The child, the family, and the marriage need both parents— especially energized and supportive parents. Anger can be directed at energizing yourself to be really active in a positive way. We discuss how to do this later in the book.

Most books on anger will tell you to find ways to reduce your anger constructively such as by exercising, going to therapy, focusing on other activities, or participating in recreation. One of the best ways is to help others. We started the first support group for families who had children with autism spectrum disorders in our area. It has enriched us and helped scores of families. We learned a great deal from the guest speakers that we invited to present to the support group and from the solutions that others have developed and shared about how they were dealing with their problems.

We have had speakers discuss diet issues, explain how the police deal with individuals with disabilities, tell about medications and treatments from a psychiatrist's perspective, and describe services provided by various support agencies. I have led discussions on the role of fathers and the importance of special needs trusts. Gena has presented on social skills training, individual education plans, and applied behavior analysis. This book is a result of those discussions and the things we have learned from other parents. God's second great commandment is to love others. What a great way to show this love by actively helping those in need and helping yourselves in the process.

You may always be a little angry and want to blame others, but this will dissipate. Long term, you will have to take some form of action in response to your situation. The most common early response is the first big D, denial. Denial is like a first line of defense against the attack on our lives and expectations. Another response is to keep going on as if nothing has changed. This is different from denial. You do not deny the existence of the disability, but you make every effort not to allow it to change your situation. You don't tell your parents, your friends, and your co-workers. This avoids embarrassment but also puts added pressure on you. This added pressure will affect you and your family and something will have to give. Frequently this will lead to increased anger and resentment.

Other Responses

Another response is to passively support your child. Some parents listen to the professionals (doctors, therapists, educators, etc.) and do what they say. This is sort of the path of least resistance because you are just following professional advice. The problem with this is that the parents know their child a lot better than any of the professionals who tend to label and classify everything in their professional language and experience but do not always know what is best for your specific child. A favorite saying in the autism community is that when you have met one person with autism, you have met one person with autism. In other words, each child is different and knowing one person with this disability does not necessarily help you understand others with similar disabilities. Each person with a disability is at least as different as each person without a disability.

> "You know your child best and you will have an intuitive knowledge of what will work and what will not work."

A final approach that you can take is the activism approach (or the active resistance approach). You know your child best and you will have an intuitive knowledge of what will work and what will not work. We made every effort to influence all of Brent's many diagnosticians and care providers. Gena was more knowledgeable much of the time, but I had an impact, too—especially on the school professionals. More on this later.

Grief

From the moment we are informed of our child's disability we are in what we call grief mode. As we discussed above, the first stage is denial. For men this can last for years! It did for this father. Denial can be a defense mechanism to give us more time to develop our inner strength to handle this new reality and to support the child with special needs and the family. This was certainly my approach for the first few years. I needed time to accept that Brent was never going to be the son I had hoped he would be. I needed time to grow up. I was 30 years old when we were first told of Brent's disability and I was not ready for this news. My character was not strong enough to look past the selfish implications of his disability. I saw the same approach from many of the men in our support group. The mothers tended to be less grief stricken and got past the denial stage much faster.

As you can see in the illustration of the ladder of grief, once we get past the total denial stage we typically get angry about the situation as discussed above. I believe that almost all of the fathers (and many mothers) in our support group were angry about the situation they found themselves in. Out of this anger can come a period when we look for ways out. Many of us will attempt to bargain with God. We offer to be better, to sacrifice time, money, or other resources if

He will just fix the problems. I know of no instances when this works—but it may be another way to buy some time for ourselves.

A very common result of getting through the first three stages is another big D, depression. Depression is a feeling of helplessness or a prolonged sense of feeling out of control and weak. We talk about this in the chapter on how to help yourself. We believe that we all get depressed from this situation at some point; it is just a matter of when, not if. Depression will usually pass after a period of time. It is important to realize that the father, the mother, and child are also very likely to be depressed at times. It is not much fun being disabled and not much fun being the primary care giver for a person with disabilities. It can be downright depressing at times.

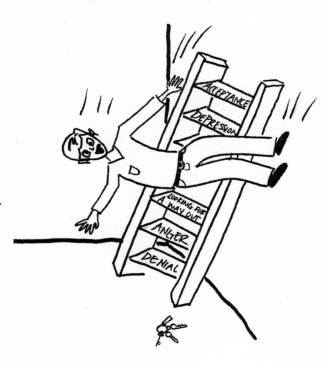

Chronic depression, on the other hand, is a much more dangerous situation that may require outside help. Chronic depression is largely caused by either a change in body chemistry or a major change in thought processes. Typically, you cannot fix this yourself in any reasonable period (months or a year or more). Sometimes it may be necessary to utilize medication to help balance the chemical situation, to have some therapeutic help, or do both. You will need to see your family doctor. Please do not be afraid to seek help.

Men rarely want to admit they are not in control. We want to be self-sufficient, to handle the situation, to be macho. So when we get depressed we try to tough it out. This can actually work for ordinary depression but can take a lot of time. Note that your family may not be too thrilled with your working through this yourself especially as it makes you less productive and it is likely you will be a lot less pleasant to be around. I am not very proud to admit that this has been my general approach for the last 25 years. Luckily I have not had chronic depression—just regular bouts of ordinary depression.

The last step of the grief process is called acceptance. But what does it mean to accept this situation? Does it mean we give up our life plans, our hopes? Does it mean we are no longer angry, do not blame anyone, and are never depressed? In fact, acceptance can be temporary. The situation may not be stable especially as the child grows and changes. It has been over 25 years for us and we are still challenged.

So what is acceptance? Does it mean we make a decision about how we will behave from now on? The bottom line answer is yes. We basically face a simple decision that has been facing us forever—either we fight or we run. This is frequently called the fight or flight option. Once we realize we will have to make major changes to deal with the situation, we have to decide to dig in and do our best or to bail out. Most fathers will initially decide to accept the challenge and do their best to support the family. However, once it appears that the situation cannot be fixed no matter how hard the father tries, it gets pretty frustrating. I have included a chapter on "Mr. Fix It" dealing with tendencies to try to solve problems. We all will consider abandoning a fight we perceive we cannot win. The solution many men consider is to leave the family and end the marriage. I discuss this critical issue in greater detail later.

> "We basically face a simple decision that has been facing us forever—either we fight or we run."

Think of the grief process as a ladder we are attempting to climb—a ladder with slippery rungs that keep shaking as in an earthquake. It is really easy to slip back to denial, to anger, into depression, or to bargaining even after we have achieved acceptance. We can be depressed and then get angry. We can be angry, and then a doctor gives us some hope from a therapy, an operation or a new drug, and we can easily slip into denial mode. We can move from acceptance when we get informed of a new problem or second ailment and quickly we get angry or depressed all over again.

The Cloud of Guilt

Accompanying grief is frequently a sense of guilt. If your child was born with a disability, it is almost impossible not to think that you had a part in causing it whether it is from your genes or behaviors prior to birth. If the disability is from an illness or from an accident, why couldn't we have done more to protect our child? Once we found out, did we do everything we could do to help? Some sense of guilt will likely be there for almost every father and mother.

People tend to be pretty rational, but guilt is really hard to rationalize away. Try as we may, there is always some sense of guilt. Guilt is a major driver of all sorts of difficulties including ruined relationships, psychological problems, and health problems. A strong sense of guilt can be disabling to yourself and can prevent you from helping with the disability and helping the family. If you are paralyzed by guilt you need to seek professional help. I know of no easy way to get rid of guilt without help. Counseling can be a great source of help. Our previous church had a grief support group that did wonderful things to help people deal with their feelings. If you have strong friendships, ask your friends to help you. Do all three if you can.

Many parents will try and ignore guilt or just live with it. Some will turn to substance abuse (also called self-medicating) to deal with the pain. The pain of guilt can lead you to depression or anger and even put you on the ladder of grief. If you want to feel even guiltier, consider the flight option above—it will cause you to feel guilty about your role in the situation and compound it with guilt about abandoning the family. This double hit of guilt can be tremendously disabling to you and may have a permanent impact on your life.

God can help you gain perspective on your situation and even provide direct help. Do not expect Him to give you special knowledge of how all of your problems will be resolved. However, having faith can give you hope, even where there seems to be no hope. Without hope, almost all parents are going to be stuck in grief and guilt. God can lead you to many people that can help you and your family.

> "Some sense of guilt will likely be there for almost every father and mother."

The most positive influence we had in our family was our local church. Virtually all of Brent's acquaintances came from the church. His social life was centered on an accepting single adult Bible study group. We had wonderful support from many members of our adult Bible study group and from the pastors. We saw many members of our support group without faith and hope, hurting with nowhere to turn. Our once per month meetings hardly helped enough; they needed more help than we could provide.

God is willing to help you if you will just have faith and ask. We have had many prayers answered in trying to help Brent. Many employers have bent rules for him. Brent once lived in a subsidized apartment and this happened almost miraculously following years of hope and prayers. One day we got a phone call that a brand new apartment complex was available that we did not even know was being built. They had reserved a unit for him! Prayer can make all the difference in the world to you and to your family.

Chapter Take-a-ways

Be realistic about your situation.

Free yourself of grief and guilt.

Be faithful to your family.

Trust God to help.

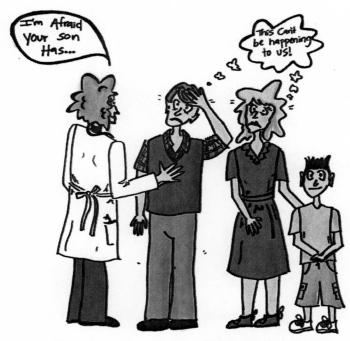

CHAPTER 2
Now What?

17

M ike is a father in his thirties who has been married to Susan for 12 years. They have two children: Jack, age 10, and Katie, age 8. Five years ago, Katie had a playground accident and banged her head on a metal pole. She now has periodic seizures and requires constant monitoring. Susan had to quit her part-time job to take care of Katie and Mike has felt increased pressure as the only financial supporter of the family. In the last two years, things have gotten worse for Katie, and Susan has had a more difficult time with problems at home and at school.

Mike and Susan have had a few intense fights about intimacy, time, and money. Mike is starting to feel less and less part of the family and is spending more hours at work. He tells Susan he needs to stay late at times in order to get ahead, but also he just doesn't really want to face coming home some nights. Susan has mentioned going to a counselor that one of her friends recommended a few times and Mike has resisted this.

Looking down the road in his life, Mike doesn't see a lot of hope for improvement. Katie seems to be stable for now, but will likely still need a lot of support for the rest of her life. Their son Jack is starting to feel resentful of all the attention Katie gets, and has started acting out at school. Mike has a shot at a job that would require traveling a day or two each week. It would mean more money and less time at home. He has started to think about his future, his career, and his marriage. He is starting to feel that something has to give. Like one of his single friends at work said the other day, "You only get one shot in this life." Mike is trying to decide which road he is going to take to get to where he thinks he wants to be.

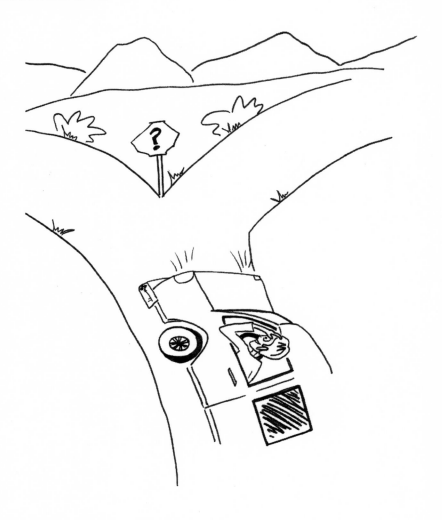

As we go down the road of life, we are constantly forced to make decisions. Many of us define ourselves by the decisions we make. When you realized that you had a child with a disability, your world changed and you were forced to start making decisions you probably did not expect to make and were probably poorly prepared to make. As discussed in the last chapter, we can deny there is a problem or pretend there is no problem, but the problem still exists.

There is pain, there is frustration, and there is a sense of unfairness. After 4 years in the Air Force and 4 years in business, I was just starting to get my business career in high gear (at least I thought so). I had just taken a management position with a food manufacturer and now I had a child with some sort of behavior problem and our daughter was going through the terrible twos. How could I stay late at work and do the little extras to get ahead when we had these problems at home? This was decision time. Each of us faces decisions, and they can be really significant to our family and to ourselves.

Some of the decisions parents make include the following:

1. What type of job can I do and still help my family?

2. How am I going to make time for my spouse and our marriage?

3. How much time can I take for myself to be with my friends, play golf, watch TV, or surf on the computer, etc.?

4. How, what, and how much am I willing to do to support the child with the disability and the rest of the family?

One way to look at some of these key decisions is by looking at life pies. Each pie represents the amount of focus, energy, and interest we have in self and in others.

Life Pie Charts

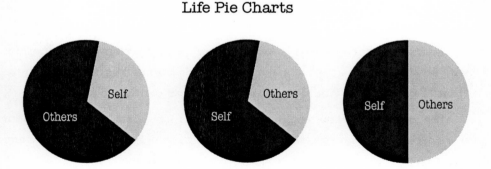

Figure 1   Figure 2   Figure 3

> "The differences between life pies 1 and 2 are not that great, but the consequences can be wonderful or tragic for you and your family."

Either we are focused on ourselves (Figure 2) or on others (Figure 1). Figure 2, in my experience, is far more common than Figure 1 with fathers. We have a career, recreation, and many activities outside of the home and family. This has completely reversed itself in our family for the last few years. Gena is a full-time professor and was the primary income provider for a brief period of time. Currently I am a distance learning professor working out of our home and we now share the role of primary income provider. With the arrival of a child with special needs many of the primary income earners will initially move from Figure 2 to Figure 3. This can be very positive and necessary. The key question is, where do we go from Figure 3? For most of us, the move to Figure 1 will be difficult and painful to our personal life goals. Many of us will want to move towards Figure 2 where we are more focused on ourselves. So back to the key question—where do we want to be? The differences between life pies 1 and 2 are not that great, but the consequences can be wonderful or tragic for you and your family.

Mike and Susan are in different life pies. Mike is a Figure 3 person with a lot of focus on his job, his family, and his personal future. Susan is a Figure 1 person with a great deal of time and energy focused on their children. Mike's new job opportunity with the travel commitment is a difficult decision. Does the family need more money or do they need more of him? What will the added pressure on Susan do to their marriage? What will be the impact on his relationships with his children? Mike could make a decision that would put him firmly in the Figure 2 category. He would be self-focused instead of other focused.

For many of us, our religious values point to Figure 1. One thing about these decisions is no matter which way we go there will be pain, difficulties, and challenges. There has never been a promise of a life without trouble.

When to Make the Big Decisions

The best time to make big decisions is to make them *before* the situation actually happens. Think about this: You made a decision to be faithful and supportive through the good times and the bad *before* you got married, right? You made the decision to be faithful and reliable to that bowling or baseball team *before* you joined, right? If you knew you were going to have a child with special needs, what better time to decide to be faithful and supportive than *before* he or she arrives? We know of a number of fathers and mothers who married into a family that had a child with a disability. They certainly made that decision before they married!

Most parents reading this book are already past the *before* option for decisions. It could be years ago that you got that diagnosis or the accident happened. You could still be in denial, anger, pleading, depression, or acceptance mode (or any combination). If you have not gotten to some level of acceptance, I urge you not to make any hasty decisions. Please read the rest of this book and digest the concepts first. If you are at a level of acceptance, then it may be time to make some decisions.

Choices and Consequences

If you have thought about leaving your family, there are several factors to consider:

1. You will radically hurt the existing family relationships between you and your children and of course with your spouse.

2. The impact on the child or the children will be more than you likely realize.

3. Placing your spouse in the position of being a single parent of a child with special needs is hard to rationalize as fair in any way to them or to your child.

4. You will likely never fully recover from this decision.

I know of no mother or father who left their family and are really happy or feel that they did the right thing. So this can be viewed as a tough lose-lose decision. If you stay, the current pain and difficulties stay, and if you leave, new pain and difficulties are created. Please read the chapter on helping yourself and the chapter on success to gain a better perspective on your decisions.

> "I know of no mother or father who left their family and are really happy or feel that they did the right thing."

Perhaps one way to look at this decision is to try to determine where you can do the most good. If you are doing more harm than good in the family because you are so angry or depressed, then some separation may be good. If you are still able to help, to provide some of the care, some respite for your spouse, help with the other children, etc., then it may be best to stay. This needs to be carefully considered by yourself, your spouse, and either close friends or professionals to get their perspectives. If separation is warranted, then it should be a temporary solution used to give you time to resolve your issues and your difficulties. Remember that marriage is a sacred commitment. God is looking out for all *His* children including you and your spouse. Permanent separation or divorce is not a good solution for any of the members of the family, unless there have been extraordinary circumstances such as abuse.

Perspective of Time

Your child, your entire family, and you are all going to grow older and change. Can you visualize what that will look like in a few years? Time is a key issue that needs to be considered. Look at time in terms of things like:

1. Goals (long-term, short-term, etc.)

2. Maturity (age as well as experience)

3. Age (yourself, your wife, and the children)

4. Vision (now, ten years from now, 25 years from now, etc.)

Maybe you have a son with autism who is 7 years old. In 10 years, science may have a cure or develop systems that allow him to live a normal life. Maybe you have a 12-year-old daughter with a crippling injury. Again, can you know what she will become as an adult? People with disabilities have dreams just as people without disabilities. These dreams for their future may be just like other's dreams or they may be very different. The point is that they have dreams and *they have a right to their dreams.*

We cannot really know the future. If we do all we can to help our child, he or she may be vastly more successful than if we do not do our best. Many fathers may be unable to help much for a while if they are in denial, but given time, they can make a difference. During the early years, I was not always helpful, but now I am more in contact with Brent than Gena is. There were times when I thought having a child with special needs was too difficult and too unfair. I wanted to escape the pain. But I made the decision early on to hang in there. The sooner you can make that decision, and make it a final decision, the better off you and your family will be!

> "People with disabilities have dreams just as people without disabilities."

A Word of Encouragement

If you don't hang in there, you won't know how much good might happen. If you do quit, you know for sure that anything that does happen will happen without you. Remember that whatever the current situation is, it will change over time. Everyone changes and who knows who will come into your life or what medical miracles will be discovered. Below is a famous short poem by an unknown author:

DON'T QUIT!

When things go wrong, as they sometimes will,
When the road you're trudging seems all uphill,

When the funds are low and the debts are high,
And you want to smile, but you have to sigh,

When care is pressing you down a bit,
Rest, if you must, but do not quit.

Life is queer with its twists and turns,
As every one of us sometimes learns,

And many a failure turns about,
When he might have won had he stuck it out;

Don't give up though the pace seems slow...
You may succeed with another blow.

Often the goal is nearer than
It seems to a faint and faltering man,

Often the struggler has given up,
When he might have captured the victor's cup,

And he learned too late when the night slipped down,
How close he was to the golden crown.

Success is failure turned inside out--
The silver tint of the clouds of doubt,

And you never can tell how close you are,
It may be near when it seems so far,

So stick to the fight when you're hardest hit--
It's when things seem worst that you must not quit.

–Author Unknown

Winston Churchill gave a famous and very short speech to the boys at Harrow School, his secondary school alma mater, in 1941:

"Never give up," he said, and returned to his seat.
He got up again. "Never give up," he said, and returned
to his seat. A third time he arose, "Never, never, in
nothing great or small, large or petty, never give in
except to convictions of honor and good sense.

Never yield to force; never yield to the apparently
overwhelming might of the enemy.
NEVER GIVE UP!" he proclaimed loudly,
and his speech was over.

There is much to be said for not giving up. Commit to a goal and stick to it, whether it be in marriage, in your work, or in taking care of a child with disabilities. These are very worthy goals. They are goals worth holding on to no matter the level of difficulty or stress. Do not let your current situation drive you to make a decision that you will regret later.

Stress Provides for Growth

Almost all of us want to grow and learn, to be better next year than we are now. If there is no stress in our lives, then we stop growing. Stress is needed to make us change, to make us try new things, to make us learn new things. Now the stress level may be pretty high with a child with special needs in the family, but is it too high? Maybe you need the stress to force you to develop your character and your strength. Will you not be of more value to your family and to your employer if you have a stronger character?

Which of us does not want to be more patient, to be able to handle a crisis better, to be the calm, sure one that others turn to when they need help? Which of us does not want to be respected for the things we have done to help others? Look at your current situation as an opportunity for growth. Hang in there and do your best, and who knows what might happen? Remember, if you leave, then whatever does happen will happen without you!

> "Look at your current situation as an opportunity for growth."

God will strengthen us and provide help to handle any situation. He cares about each of us and will be there for us. Thousands of years ago He made a promise:

> So do not fear, for I am with you;
>
> do not be dismayed, for I am your God.
>
> I will strengthen you and help you;
>
> I will uphold you with my righteous right hand (Isaiah 41:10 NIV).

Bad things happen to both good people and bad people. The difference is how we respond. Make good decisions that make sense for all concerned and for the long term, not just for how things look right now. Who knows how great a person you can become given enough stress, enough push to change and grow? Who knows how successful your spouse, your family, and your children will be if you just do your best?

> "Bad things happen to both good people and bad people. The difference is how we respond."

Chapter Take-a-ways:

The future may be brighter than the present.

Make decisions with a long-term perspective.

Don't quit!

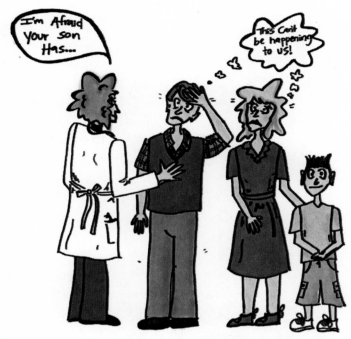

CHAPTER 3
A Father's Perspective

31

I will never forget one of the first parent-teacher conferences we attended when Brent was in Kindergarten. We already had been informed that Brent was one of a group of children that was at risk for being unsuccessful in school. The whole team was there: the school social worker, counselor, school psychologist, and learning disabilities specialist. They seemed to be unsure of themselves and their recommendations were pretty much a soft sell except for the psychologist. He had some strong Freudian ideas about Brent's problems. We did not accept his ideas and he quickly backed down. I believe my presence in the meeting prevented him from pushing this and the team from being overly aggressive with their recommendations.

As a father, you have a unique role to play in the life of your family, and this is even more important to a family with a child with a disability. The father is typically:

1. The protector of the family
2. The supporter of his spouse
3. The key provider
4. The role model for how a man is expected to behave
5. The leader of the family
6. A family member who has unique capabilities

These roles are carried out in the home, in the school, socially, and in employment. The provider role often means the father is outside the home most days leaving the wife to deal with the daily problems. In addition to the above unique roles, the father is also the backup to the mother. Whenever the wife is unable to take care of the family, the father needs to be ready and able to fill the gap.

In the School

In the school setting, the father's attendance at an IEP (Individual Education Plan) meeting can be very powerful. Most IEP meetings consist of a 3-5 member education specialist team typically talking with the mother. It is very hard for one person to understand all the proposals and analysis being presented by a number of different specialists. The father's presence can enhance the chances of the couple understanding what is being proposed. I attended a number of Brent's IEP meetings and believe that I presented unique questions that the team was not used to considering. This led to some revisions in their approach.

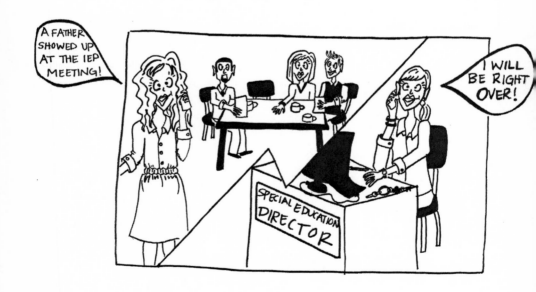

Frequently a father's presence will change the entire tone of the meeting. It is not too hard for an education team to convince one person they have the best approach, but having a second person makes it much more likely that all the child's needs will be addressed. Plus, the father adds a second person listening and this may tend to make the education team more careful of what they say.

> "A father's involvement can be essential in making sure that his child and wife are treated properly and receive the services they need."

A father's involvement can be essential in making sure that his child and wife are treated properly and receive the services they need. There is a significant portion of the population that will respond much better to a man than to a woman. For example, there are an increasing number of doctors, technicians, and specialists from overseas living and working in the United States. The role of women in some of the countries which these providers come from is significantly limited and some of these service providers may have an inherent bias. Your presence in meetings with these people can make a huge difference in how seriously they respond to your family's needs. I have firsthand knowledge of how well this works in a number of meetings I have attended. A father's presence adds strength to most interactions with school personnel.

Protector of the Family

Many people will not be comfortable around your child with a disability. They will feel awkward and may not know what to say or how to act. Other children may be especially cruel making fun of your child in school and in the neighborhood. With some disabilities, other children will take advantage of your child's need to be accepted into the group. This is especially true of disabilities like autism, Asperger Syndrome, and other developmental disorders where your child does not really understand social situations well and wants to be accepted.

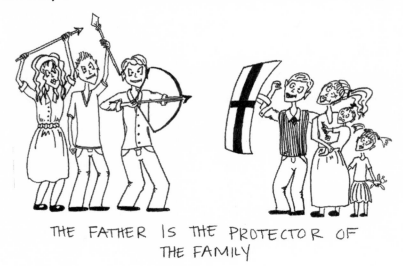

THE FATHER IS THE PROTECTOR OF THE FAMILY

Support Your Wife in Promoting Socialization

Remember that your child will likely have the same desires as other children to have friends, to play, to have common interests with other children, and to want to wear the latest styles to fit in with peers. So what does a father do to help? The first thing is to support your wife's efforts. Gena did many things to help Brent socialize. We had many young people over to our house or out to the movies with us to attempt to help Brent feel he had friends. We had birthday parties with the neighborhood children and Gena invited other children to go to many activities with our family.

Do everything you can to create places where you child is accepted. You can be involved in 4H or Girl Scouts. You can help your son join Boy Scouts (or similar organizations) and go on campouts and other activities with him. I was a Weeblo leader (the year between Cub Scouts and Boy Scouts) for a year to help facilitate the social interactions Brent needed. We went on a number of campouts together. The whole family spent four summers at a church camp where Gena was an age group director and I volunteered on weekends. Our two children had a wonderful time as two of the camp kids. I also taught Sunday school for his grade one year. This was a challenge because Brent's attention span was very short and he tended to disrupt the class. Your children will need your help in developing social relationships. Attending church and organizational activities like the YMCA are a great way to make this happen. We have found that larger churches may have more program options that you can take advantage of. Frequently you do not even need to be a church member to be involved in many of these activities.

Educate Others

Perhaps the best thing you can do to help your child is to educate the adults and the other children in organizations your child wants to join. They will tend to treat your child differently if they do not understand the disability out of fear of saying or doing something wrong. Education is especially needed for the developmental, emotional and other disabilities that are not visible. I had talks with leaders in Little League, in karate, school band, etc. Your wife may be able to do a lot of these talks, but frequently the father has a unique effectiveness in these situations. Gena was much more active than I was in educating others about Brent for most of his school

> "Perhaps the best thing you can do to help your child is to educate the adults and the other children in organizations your child wants to join."

years. However, as I increased my involvement in a variety of settings, Gena and I were able to work together as a team to help Brent. We saw better outcomes as Brent was accepted into groups. This effort continues to this day.

When a child is old enough to work, the father has a similar role to play with employers. Again, I have had many meetings with Brent's bosses over the years.

Employers will tend to be accommodating if they understand what is needed. A father who identifies with the business concerns of an employer will often be able to intervene using the language of business and management that makes sense to an employer. This usually holds true whether the employer is male or female.

In early 2005 Brent was having difficulty with a co-worker who had a strong personality. Brent called in sick twice to avoid the situation. The worker had no authority, but wanted things done his way and he intimidated Brent. I met with Brent's boss and Brent, and we talked about how good the other worker was, but that Brent felt intimidated by him and questioned his role in telling Brent what to do at work. The boss cleared up the situation by assigning each employee a different area of responsibility, which suited Brent just fine. Brent did not know how to talk to the boss without making negative remarks about the other employee. My intervention as an advocate for Brent led to a positive outcome.

I have had to push myself to do these meetings at times. When I have avoided talking to employers, Brent has had trouble. These meetings may be easy for you to do. However, if it is hard, remember, you, the father, are likely the best advocate for your child. Sometimes your child may not want you to "interfere." Brent has told us many times that things are fine. One time this was just days before he got fired! Many workers with special needs do not know when there are problems brewing, and an extra effort by you, even an intrusive effort, may make the difference between keeping the job or losing it. If you are unsure about whether or not to get involved in an employment situation, err to the side of over-involvement.

Father as Provider

One of the major frustrations of the father is being the major provider, and in many cases the only provider of money for the family. The extra needs of a child with a disability can frequently prevent a wife from working full-time or even part-time. The result is that the father has to do it all. But there is more. There may be many extra costs that occur for a child with a disability. These will surely include paying all the deductibles for your insurance, but may also include paying for treatments, medications, or equipment that insurance does not cover. You may want to pay for a specialist that is not "in your medical plan" or try a treatment that is not accepted as common practice by the insurance company. You will likely have to buy the most expensive insurance option at work to cover more of your child's special needs.

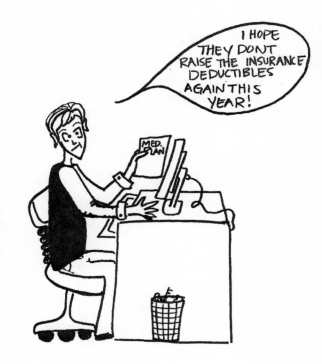

On top of all this, the type of job that you need to support your child usually must include a decent benefit package. If you have dreamed of owning your own business (as many do), you may have to put that off indefinitely. Working for an exciting start-up company may not be workable. Insurance for a small business will not likely work once the insurance company realizes the costs they will have to incur to support your child. The insurance company will often raise rates to cover all of that cost. A larger employer can prevent higher insurance costs because the insurance carrier has to charge the same rates for all of the employees. Your additional costs are balanced by the large pool of other employees that do not have high medical costs. It may be wise to make sure you have good disability coverage in case you cannot work, and sufficient life insurance to cover at least four to five times your annual pay. These are all additional costs you might not have otherwise.

Father as Role Model

As the male role model for the family, the father carries a responsibility to, among other things, handle stress, provide for the needs of the family, and show tenderness to those he loves. The way the father carries out his responsibilities will deeply affect what his children perceive as "normal." By following a basic blueprint of leadership, the leader of the home can say to those who follow him not only "Do as I say," but "Do as I do." Remember that children will model what they observe in the home. They will choose their recreation, language, friends, and habits related to what they see and hear. Everything you do will be a model for your children.

> "Remember that children will model what they observe in the home."

One of the roles that is very important is supporting your partner. No father has all the answers and many times the other partner has a better solution to a problem or a situation. The father that is strong enough in character to acknowledge when his partner is right and he is wrong is a great model for others to see. While the father may be the final decision maker, a wise father will listen before he decides. Gena frequently had better intuition and better approaches than I did. Some of my best decisions were to follow her suggestions instead of my own. In the family with a child that has special needs, this is of significant importance. Most likely, your partner knows your children better than you do. She spends more time with them than you do. She sees who their friends are and how others treat your child. I urge you to follow her lead unless you are absolutely certain that your approach is better. A strong but humble father is a great role model for his family and also for those outside of the family.

Father as Leader of the Family

In most societies including our own, the father is the head of the household. As such, he has the responsibility for the overall welfare of each member and for the family as a whole. He is called to guide and discipline his children and he is empowered to make final decisions for the good of all members of the family. These responsibilities are clearly more challenging for a family with a child with a disability. You will be judged by the way you handle these responsibilities and by the decisions you make for the good of the family. The true story by Carl Catt in this book is a wonderful example of a father who took on the responsibilities he felt he needed to do and the great and selfless decisions he made.

Using Capabilities

The father is obviously in a unique position in the family. He is the leader and many times the final decision maker. He is usually the main provider and a role model for the family. The father is the protector of the family and he is usually the physically strongest person in the family. Usually he is the one that kills the wasp in the bedroom and shovels the driveway when it snows. He fixes the leaky faucet, keeps the car running, and builds the playhouse in the back yard. He does the taxes and helps the children learn algebra. He gets up early on Saturday to mow the lawn and fixes the flat tire on the bike.

In some families, other people accomplish many of these functions. This can be because the mother is very capable of doing the taxes or killing wasps. Also it can also be because the grandfather or neighbors come over to mow the lawn or fix the car. A primary reason that others do these functions is because the father is not there to do them. The father needs to be there to use his capabilities. As we discussed in the previous chapter, this is a key decision that needs to be made. The most capable father is not worth much if he is not there when he is needed.

The Primary Caregiver Role

There are quite a few fathers that have taken on the role of primary caregiver for their child with a disability. Some fathers have lost their wives to illness or injury or the wife has left the family for personal reasons. Whatever the reason, the father now also has the tasks that the wife did in the past. Housekeeping, cooking, transportation, accompanying the child to the doctors and therapists and many other tasks are now left for the father. I have some familiarity with this situation as Gena was the primary income earner for a while and I worked at home during this period of time. I certainly gained a better understanding of what it takes to keep up a house! We hired a cleaner to do the vacuuming, dusting, and kitchen and bathroom cleaning every other week. Gena did those chores for the first 34 years of our marriage. I did not do them well, and so we hired the professionals.

I firmly believe that the caregiver role is of primary importance in the eyes of God. Taking care of those with a disability and in need is a most honorable role to play. It is certainly not an easy role and many in our society do not lift it up as something to strive for. I firmly believe that the trials we face are God's way of helping us grow. A father taking on the primary caregiver role is a challenge. Out of this challenge can come growth and new understandings of what is important to God. Not many of us will gain new abilities, skills, and knowledge unless challenged to do so. God may have put you right where he wants you for your own good and for the good of others. If you are the primary caregiver, know that this is honorable and worthy. If you are not the primary caregiver, then honor the person who is. Support that person in every way you can for the good of the family, the children, and the marriage.

Chapter Take-a-ways:

You are the leader of the family.

You are a unique asset to your family.

Use your capabilities to strengthen your family.

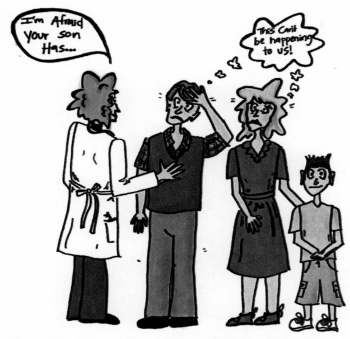

CHAPTER 4
A Mother's Perspective

43

Discussing this book with Press as he was writing it gave me the oppor-tunity to reflect on my perspective as the mother of a son with special needs. My perspective may be different from yours, and it is certainly different from Press's. However, I do believe that there is value in sharing our perspectives because it can help others realize that they are not alone in facing life's many challenges, and we can learn from each other's experiences. If I can make someone else's journey in life a little easier by sharing suggestions and lessons I have learned, then I will have fulfilled my task in writing this chapter.

It is amazing to me to realize that Press and I have experienced many of the same situations and dilemmas as Brent's parents, and yet, we did not always react in the same manner or experi-ence the opportunities

> "...there is value in sharing our perspectives because it can help others realize that they are not alone in facing life's many challenges, and we can learn from each other's experiences."

presented to us in the same way. For the first 33 years of our marriage, Press provided most of the financial resources for our family, and he worked outside of the home. I was a homemaker, part-time worker, full-time worker, and gradu-ate student at various times over those 33 years, as well as the glue that held the family together and made sure everyone got to their appointments, etc. During the last 3 years I have worked full-time outside of the home as a college professor teaching courses in special education and autism. Press has been working mostly from home as a college distance learning program professor. He has taken over my former role of the day-to-day overseeing of Brent and he makes sure that Brent gets to doctor appointments, etc. We have virtually switched parenting roles and it has been extremely eye opening! It also has reminded us again that we are definitely wired differently! Fortunately, we have been able to work together as a team, although it has not always been smooth, and certainly not easy. For the majority of the difficult situations, one of us was able to shoulder the challenges Brent presented when the other one was not up to it. However, there were times when we both became discouraged and felt worn out and ready to throw in the towel. Perhaps these were the times God used to help us remember to rely on Him and seek Him personally as well as seek Him through relationships with others who could spiritually and emotionally support us.

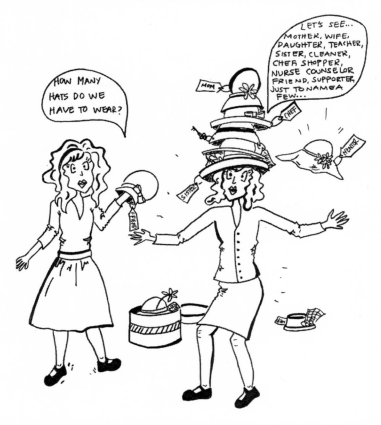

As women, we wear many hats and are involved in many different relationships. We may be wives, sisters, sister-in-laws, daughters, daughter-in-laws, nieces, granddaughters, grandmothers, aunts, cousins, friends, homemakers, employees, students, teachers, counselors, mentors and advocates, just to name a few. All of these roles influence how we view our parenting role. As women we tend to place a high importance on relationships to define us. Therefore, when Press originally asked me to write a chapter on the importance of mothers, I was torn as to how to separate this role from the many relationships that characterize my life. I cannot satisfactorily separate these roles; therefore, I will present the lessons I have learned because of my relationships. The following important lessons I learned will be discussed in the chapter:

1. There are numerous positives associated with having a child with a disability. It gives us an opportunity to learn lessons, gain new perspectives, and meet people that we may not have had the chance to know if we did not have a child with a disability.

2. Trust your intuition as a mother. Parents truly do know their children better than anyone else, except God.

3. It is important to seek support from other women.

4. Many women tend to be nurturers and want someone to listen to them as they share concerns, while the men in their lives tend to try to be "fixers" and want to solve problems. Sometimes we just want to be heard and we are not asking for problems to be fixed. Furthermore, not all problems can be fixed.

5. God will give us other people to help encourage us.

6. Healing does not necessarily mean God will take away your child's disability. Healing may occur in another area of your life such as a restored relationship or the beginning of a deeper spiritual relationship.

7. It is important to take time for respite, rest, and relaxation for your mental health as well as the mental health of the family. Slowing down has not been easy for me! This may involve spending some time alone, time with other women, and time to nurture your marriage or significant relationships.

You Say There Are Positives
in Raising a Child with a Disability?

Press and I had been very focused on the importance of academics and on achieving academic success. Probably the fact that we are both first-born children and are both competitive added to this conviction. When Brent began having learning problems early in his school life, we began to realize that academics might not be as important as we once thought they were. Brent's academic struggles began to cause us to reevaluate our priorities and values and to contemplate the meaning of success. This did not happen overnight and it did not happen without first going through many challenging times. It took us a long time to realize that our expectations needed to change and that Brent was not going to fit into the same mold that we had. Furthermore, his successes were going to be very different from ours. We did invest a lot of time during Brent's childhood exposing him to various activities (e.g., karate, Cub Scouts, playing the trumpet, etc.) so that he could determine what he liked and was good at. We hoped that we could help him by capitalizing on his strengths.

Facilitating a support group of 350 families of children with autism spectrum disorders gave us the blessed opportunity to hear about others' joys and struggles in parenting. Many parents told us that their child taught them patience and that they would not have been the same individuals if they had not had the experience of raising their child. They became stronger, more confident, and learned how to be advocates for their children's needs. I know that Brent has helped us to see the world in a different way. We learned to value differences and celebrate others' unique qualities. If it was not for Brent, I would not be in the profession that I am in and I probably would not have devoted my time and career to helping and teaching others about children with special needs. I also probably would not have had the opportunity to get to know many of the individuals with special needs and their families that I met if it was not for Brent. These people have enriched my life and have helped support us through some challenging situations. I have to say that Brent's uncanny ability to "think outside the box" has certainly provided us with a fresh new outlook.

In *The Soul of Autism*, William Stillman (2008) describes additional positive benefits of raising a child with an autism spectrum disorder (ASD) that were shared with him by parents during consultations they requested for assistance. Some parents stated that their parenting experience humbled them; another parent stated that it gave her courage beyond words and she no longer felt intimidated; and other parents stated that they gained patience and learned to value things they ignored in the past. Others shared that they were now less selfish and that having a child with special needs made them look to a Higher Power and to learn the true meaning of love. Another parent said that it helped her to grow up, while another parent said that she learned that nothing was impossible with God. Still another parent commented that she saw a better side of humanity as she watched parents prevail through many obstacles to get their child the services he or she needed and that she personally had to become a better and more efficient housekeeper in order to keep some of life's chaos under control.

I was particularly struck by the comment that one parent made in saying that she realized that she was not in control as she experienced challenges raising her child with special needs. I believe that God has given me numerous opportunities to learn this lesson as well. In fact, I continue to struggle with this lesson. I find it very comforting to know that God has asked us to turn our troubles over to Him and that we do not have to carry the worries of the world on our shoulders. I truly thought that many of the experiences I faced, both good and bad, were under my control and that if I just tried harder I could make difficult situations better. In fact, I operated under this erroneous belief for most of my life. It was not until I was faced with overwhelming anxiety and depression that I realized that I cannot control my life and that I never could. In fact, God does not want that! What a relief it was to realize that we are not supposed to be in control of our lives and that God is walking with us and carrying our burdens. Unfor-

> "God has asked us to turn our troubles over to Him... we do not have to carry the worries of the world on our shoulders."

tunately, I find that I continually try to take back my burdens, even though I know this is not right. I am making my life more complicated than it needs to be when I try to be in control. I need to remind myself to listen to Twila Paris's song *"God Is in Control"* so that I can refocus on what is truly important and what God wants me to do versus what I think I need to do.

Trust Your Intuition as a Mother

You may have faced some challenges dealing with medical professionals or educational professionals during the diagnostic evaluation of your child or in trying to obtain services to assist your child in his or her activities of daily living, including schooling. We certainly did! I hope that your experiences were positive and you felt respected by the professionals. Unfortunately, this is not always the case. When you find yourself in an encounter that is not respectful, do not give up hope or resign yourself to believing that the professionals are the "experts" and they must, therefore, know more than you. They may be the experts in their specific area of training, but they are not the experts on *your child*. Parents truly know their children

> "Parents truly know their children better than anyone else, except God."

better than anyone else, except God. Do not be intimidated by professionals who use jargon and hard to understand language, demand that you do what they say is best for your child, try to avoid talking with you, or act dismissive of your comments. I felt intimidated many times when I sat in Brent's IEP (Individual Education Plan) meetings at school and it was me and Press, or sometimes just me, and eight or more educational professionals sitting across the table.

When I train teachers now, I share my experiences as a parent and tell them what I learned about how it feels to sit on "the other side of the table." It was quite a different experience for me attending IEP meetings as a professional and helping plan educational programs for students than it was attending them as Brent's mother. I believe that educators (of which I am one, too!) need to put themselves in the shoes of the parents they work with and try to interact with them the way they would want to be treated if the roles were reversed. I also explain to teachers the importance of working collaboratively with parents and the need to help parent(s) feel comfortable and valued at their child's educational planning meetings. After all, they are the true experts on their child and they will be his or her parents for life, while we may only be their teacher for one or several years. I suggest that the educators make contact with their students' parents as soon as possible at the beginning of the new school year to open the lines of communication; introduce themselves to the parents and shake their hands when the parent or parents arrive at the school; and share positive comments about the student first before discussing the problems and challenges. Furthermore, the teacher who works the most with the child needs to sit near the parents and not on the other side of the room so that the parents do not feel that they are outnumbered by many experts at the table.

The pediatricians that I worked for as a Registered Nurse (I was a nurse prior to becoming an educator, counselor, and school psychologist) were respectful to me when I came into the office as Brent's mother. That was not always the case when I came into the office as one of their nurses. However, when I was in the role of Brent's mother they tried to reassure me that everything was okay and not to worry. I knew intuitively that something was not right, but it was hard to describe and pinpoint. They quickly reminded me that Brent was reaching his developmental milestones within the normal age expectations, even though he was at the late end of the normal expectations. They also said that sometimes boys are slower in their development than girls are. In looking back on this situation, I believe that they thought they were providing me the best advice they could and they were trying to allay my anxiety. However, this is a typical pattern that occurs with children with developmental delays. According to First Signs (2003), 70% of children with developmental delays, such as autism and Asperger Syndrome, are not identified by their pediatricians. Telling parents to

"Wait and see" or "He's just a boy and boys develop slower than girls" are typical responses given to mothers' concerns, and it just delays the diagnosis. Getting an early diagnosis is important so that interventions can be implemented as soon as possible to help the child.

We had many other encounters with medical professionals since that time and sometimes we were treated with respect and asked for our opinion and at other times we were not treated with respect. One doctor indicated that I seemed to be too involved in Brent's life. He also misdiagnosed Brent, so I think that he may not have been as involved as he should have been in order to make the correct diagnosis! What I learned from all of these experiences is that I need to trust my instincts and not let others try to convince me otherwise. Sometimes medical professionals have a difficult time admitting that they do not know how to cure a condition or that they cannot save a person from a terminal illness. Perhaps these professionals have control issues, as I do, and that may be why they tend to avoid people they cannot help or blame the person and his mother for the lack of improvement. I did come to realize that God gave me the gift of discernment and I needed to use it to advocate for my child.

The Importance of Other Women

Cultivating friendships with other girls as I grew up and with other women when I became an adult has been an important part of my life. I continued to place a high value on friendships with other women when I married, but I also naively thought that Press should fulfill *all* of my emotional needs. After all, he was my husband and isn't that what husbands are supposed to do? I don't know how I came to believe that, but I held fast to it during our early married years. Of course this lead to disappointment when I realized that Press could not do this for me. In fact, I was telling him late one evening when Brent and Kristen were young children about my concerns with Brent and about my many worries, including the realization that I had past hurts from my childhood, and Press asked me to find a girlfriend to share these things with because he just could not handle any more of my burdens. I had been frequently sharing my personal disappointments and my concerns about Brent at this time because he was having significant challenges and I did not know what to do. I felt like I

> "...women react to stress with brain chemicals that cause them to make friendships with other women."

had been kicked in the stomach when Press firmly made this request and also said that he needed to get some sleep. In other words, the conversation was over for the night! I remember also feeling cheated because Press was not fulfilling his role as my husband; I should say the role I thought he should have. What I did not realize was that Press was also struggling with challenges at his job that he kept to himself and his plate was full! Press was a lot better at compartmentalizing problems than I was. This actually may have been one of the best requests Press made of me because it jolted me to reevaluate my needs and my relationships. I did come to realize that no one person can fulfill all of another person's needs. Although I still consider Press to be my best friend after 36 years of marriage, I still need the friendships of other women.

Gale Berkowitz (2005) reported that a UCLA study on friendships among women suggested women react to stress with brain chemicals that cause them to make friendships with other women. In other words, women do not necessarily only react to stress with flight or fight reactions as was once thought. This study reportedly indicated that when women befriended other women more oxytocin was released, which lead to a calming effect. It is interesting to note that most of the previous research on stress had been conducted on males, and they produce testosterone in reaction to stress, which diminishes the effects of oxytocin. Drs. Klein and Taylor of the UCLA study developed the concept of "tend and befriend" and suggested that this may be why women live longer than men. Berkowitz (2005) also highlighted the results of the Nurses' Health Study conducted at Harvard University that revealed the more friends women had, the more likely they were to lead an enjoyable life and the less likely they were to develop physical illnesses as they became older.

Sister Joan Chittister, the author of *The Friendship of Women: The Hidden Tradition of the Bible*, stated,

> I consider friendship to be a social sacrament, a sacred act far above and beyond 'connections,' acquaintanceship, or the neighborliness of social contracts. The ability to sustain friendships is a factor in mental health, in personal development, and in emotional survival (Frietas, 2006).

Developmental psychology books describe women's friendships as involving more closeness, intimacy and self-disclosure than men's friendships. In fact, women typically have more friends than men. Men tend to do activities together and women tend to talk together and provide emotional support for each other. Moen (1996), as cited in Boyd and Bee (2006), indicated that women frequently fill the role of kin-keeper, which means that they are in charge of sustaining family and friendship relationships. They write the letters, make the phone calls, and orchestrate the get-togethers for family and friends. Women, therefore, fulfill more of a relationship role than men do. Boyd and Bee tell us that in almost all cultures women are responsible for maintaining the emotional characteristics of relationships with family, friends, and their children. I have been fortunate to have friendships with women who have sustained me emotionally throughout my adult life. Since we have moved to five different states over the last 36 years, I am not able to see some of the friends I made as often as I would like; however, they are only a phone call or an email away. We may not have talked for some time and yet we seem to be able to pick up right where we left off, even if years have passed before we're able to reconnect.

Just Listen to Me, You Don't Need to Fix It

Oftentimes the best thing anyone can do for me when I am hurting is to just listen and allow me to vent my hurts, fears, and frustrations. This involves a willingness on the listener's part to feel okay with not having the answers to help me solve whatever problem I am facing. When I was studying to be a counselor, one of the first lessons we learned was to reflect the counselee's feelings. Instead of providing platitudes such as "It's going to be alright," we were to paraphrase what they said and be nonjudgmental, open, and honest so that the counselee could continue to explore his or her beliefs, attitudes, values, behaviors, and feelings. In other words, we were facilitators, not the problem solvers. In this safe and supportive counseling environment the counselee would develop self-understanding and understanding of others so that he or she could decide on a course of action.

In *Men Are from Mars, Women Are from Venus,* Gray (1992) wrote, "A woman under stress is not immediately concerned with finding solutions to her problems but rather seeks relief by expressing herself and being understood" (p. 36). Furthermore he stated that men who are stressed tend to focus on one problem and put other problems aside while women under stress tend to become flooded by all problems. Women tend to feel better when they discuss all of their troubles—past, present, future, and potential troubles. The more they are able to express these issues and explore them, the better they feel. Gray then asserted, "To expect otherwise is to deny a woman a sense of herself" (p. 36). However, men tend to avoid listening to women talking about their problems because they believe she is either holding him responsible or blaming him for her troubles, or she wants advice. Moreover, "Just as a man is fulfilled working out the intricate details of solving a problem, a woman is fulfilled through talking about the details of her problem" (Gray, 1992, p. 39).

God Will Give Us Other People to Provide Encouragement

I was fortunate to be able to meet girlfriends who lived out of town for an overnight visit to shop and talk when my children were young. These "girlfriend breaks" provided much needed refreshment and support. When I was unable to continue my "girlfriend breaks," God provided other ways for me to receive nurture and support from others. Sometimes this support came from our couples' Bible study, a new acquaintance at work, a women's Bible study, a walking buddy, my cousin, my mother, or a new friend at school and work. The phone was a very important line of communication for me when our children were young. I met my friend Alyce at graduate school and we lived about 15 miles apart. She lived in another county and had a different telephone area code. We would always laugh when we were reminded that we were able to talk to each other for hours for free. This was in the 1980s before free cell phone coverage and another area code almost always meant expensive long-distance charges from a land phone line. We used to say that someone must have known our need to talk on the phone for this connection to be free for us. On school snow days we spent a lot of time talking on the phone if we could not meet in person. I have not seen Alyce for several years and our phone conversations are much fewer and farther between; however, we plan to catch up in a few weeks when I will spend just 24 hours with her. I imagine we will stay up very late trying to catch up where we left off and maximize our short time together.

When we lived in the Kansas City area, several of the people in our Bible study group were a good support system for us. They told us that although they did not always understand what we were going through, they would pray for us and continue to encourage us. It eventually became apparent to us who we could and could not trust with some of the painful experiences we faced. We were surprised and hurt a few times when church members or staff would disclose something that we thought we had shared with them in confidence. I imagine that this especially hurt since we tended to hold church people to a higher standard and then were disappointed when they did not meet that standard. My friends at work were especially helpful to me during this time. We all worked in the area of special education, so perhaps we were more accepting of others' differences and it made it easier to share information that others might not so readily understand.

Healing Does Not Mean
The Disability Will Be Removed

Oftentimes we pray for a cure for our child's disability and we may be very disappointed when the cure or healing does not happen in the way that we requested. This does not mean that God is not listening to us. It may mean that what we asked for is not in our best interest or in our child's best interest. It also may mean that God has different timing. He may be trying to show us something that we would never have the opportunity to see if it was not for the disability. To be honest, I cannot say that I always was comforted knowing that God's timing was not the same as my timing or that perhaps he was trying to show me something in the midst of this affliction. There were times when I wanted to be in control and just have this situation resolved NOW! I think that this is partly because I had different expectations and plans than God had for me. Expectations have probably been at the root of most of my disappointments. Expectations of what a good friend should be, a family member should be, and even what my husband should be have let me down when they did not act as I had expected. They also had their own issues and struggles that impacted how they acted. Perhaps they were scared and did not know how to react in some situations. God's message to lean on him is so simple and yet we complicate it by trying to take back the control of our lives instead of leaving it up to Him to handle.

I have been privileged to see some people find healing in other areas of their lives when they were asking for a physical healing for a loved one. Healing for one friend came in the form of more intimacy in the marriage relationship well before a physical healing became evident. Seeing this convinced me that I do not know what to pray for, but God does. I want to pass this mes-

> "God's message to lean on him is so simple and yet we complicate it by trying to take back the control of our lives instead of leaving it up to Him to handle."

sage on so that others might be encouraged that healing may well be taking place and it may be even better than we could have imagined or have known to ask for.

I do not believe that acceptance of our child's disability is something that we strive for and once we have attained it the rest of life is smooth sailing. I think we experience our loss in stages similar to the stages of death and dying that Dr. Kubler-Ross described, even when our child does not have a terminal illness but rather a chronic condition. These stages also are not linear. We can move back and forth in each stage. We may have accepted our child's diagnosis and then later find ourselves at one of the earlier stages of grief such as bargaining with God or feeling angry again. When Brent first was diagnosed by the school team in first grade as Neurologically Impaired, I was in denial. We continued to go to specialists to look for answers, but no one was sure what Brent had at that time. There were certainly times of depression in the years that followed. When Brent experienced success in high school, I thought that he had finally compensated for some of his learning challenges and that he would experience a positive future and find his place in this world. These expectations were dashed when he crashed during his college years and needed to be hospitalized for a suicide attempt. I later began doing some research and came upon the diagnosis of Asperger Syndrome. I was sure that this explained all of the inconsistencies and challenges that Brent had been facing. When this diagnosis was finally confirmed by a psychologist just before Brent's 22nd birthday, I was tremendously relieved. Right after the relief, I started to feel very sad because the reality that this was a life-long condition became apparent. The sadness did not last long, but it was definitely there. But wait a minute, I was supposed to be feeling acceptance! After all, I was the one who found the diagnosis and then went to the professionals for confirmation. Surely, I was not surprised by the diagnosis. I believe that the sadness that I was experiencing was part of the normal grief process.

Schedule Respite Time!

Getting some time away from the day-to-day challenges can provide the refreshment and relaxation that we need to come back and face the challenges of raising a child with a disability with renewed energy. In addition to the occasional "girlfriend breaks" I took, Press and I would schedule time to go on "dates" with each other during our marriage. It may sound silly, but it was too easy to get so busy that we would not have time for each other, so we decided to schedule short breaks for an evening or afternoon out when we could get a babysitter. We also switched babysitting with friends a few times in order to have some time away. I would watch their children for two days and they would watch mine for two days. It was hard for me to ask others to help me (remember my control issues!), so we did not do this often.

My mother-in-law also volunteered to watch Brent and Kristen at her home when Press had to travel to California for a business trip that I was invited to join. The children were both young then and neither attended school yet. When I came home after being gone five days, my mother-in-law emphatically stated that she now had a true appreciation of what I went through on a daily basis. We did not even realize at this time that Brent had a disability. Little did any of us know that later life would become significantly more challenging.

Spending time alone with the siblings of the child with a disability is also important. I took Kristen on some short trips and outings so that we could have time alone away from her brother. I even took her on one of my "girlfriend breaks," but she did not have as much fun as she thought she would. Kristen commented that she could not understand what was so fun about these "girlfriend breaks." I

> "Getting some time away from the day-to-day challenges can provide the refreshment and relaxation that we need to come back and face the challenges of raising a child with a disability with renewed energy."

wish I would have found some other creative ways to help Kristen to feel special. She did seem to get short changed on attention when Brent was having so many challenges that had to be dealt with immediately.

One of my graduate students asked me recently in class what I would have done differently if I had known that Brent had Asperger Syndrome when he was a child. I am not sure that my parenting would have been that much different. I would have liked to have had more patience. However, I was able to change my typically reactive approach to a calmer approach when dealing with my children's behavior over time after learning about these skills in my counseling courses. Having a diagnosis would have helped us to understand that Brent had a neurological condition that caused him to behave differently and that most of his behavior was not manipulative and volitional, even though it appeared that way. It might have helped his sister to know this and to know that he was not purposely trying to embarrass her. Most of all I wish that I would have known that we were not alone in raising Brent. There were other parents just like us who were also keeping many of their hurts private. But most importantly, I did not turn over all my anxiety to God as He asks us to do. He was always walking beside us in the good times and the bad times and I was too anxiety ridden to even realize that. Don't let your worries rob you of the joy in life that you were meant to experience.

> "Don't let your worries rob you of the joy in life that you were meant to experience."

Chapter Take-a-ways:

Don't go through this journey alone.

You can grow from this experience.

Nourish your relationships.

Turn your burdens over to God.

References

Berkowitz, G. (2005). UCLA study on friendship among women. *Women's Digest*.

    Retrieved from http://www.womensdigest.net/departments/healfit/hf0505d.html

Boyd, D., & Bee, H. (2006). *Lifespan development* (4th ed.). Boston: Pearson Education.

First Signs. (2003). *On the spectrum: Children and autism* video. First Signs.

Freitas, D. (May 3, 2006). Interview with Joan Chittister. *Religious Bookline - Publishers Weekly*.

    Retrieved from http://donnafreitasinterviews.blogspot.com/2006/07/joan-chittister-friendship-of-women.html

Gray, J. (1992). *Men are from Mars, women are from Venus: A practical guide for improving communication and getting what you want in your relationships*. New York: HarperCollins.

Moen, P. (1996). Gender, age, and the life course. In R. H. Binstock & L. K. George (Eds.), *Handbook of aging and the social sciences* (4th ed., pp. 171-187). San Diego, CA: Academic Press.

Stillman, W. (2008). *The soul of autism*. Franklin Lakes, NJ: Career Press.

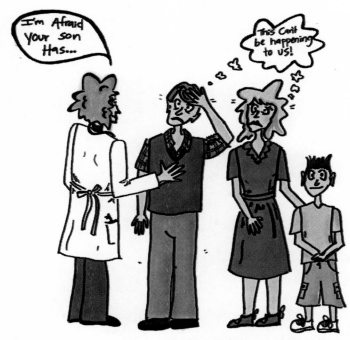

CHAPTER 5
Strains on the Marriage

63

Our marriage has faced many of the same strains that are found in most marriages. The grass has looked greener in other places, especially during times of high stress and strain. We have disagreed on issues of how to spend our time and over concerns regarding intimacy and control. We are both first-born children with two younger siblings and we were accustomed to getting our way. We both had fathers that were not as supportive as was needed and mothers that tried their best to pick up the slack. We also had a son with a significant disability. We did not have it easy, but we stuck together.

The statistics for marriages staying together are pretty grim. For families with a child with special needs there have been reports that up to 80% of families have divorced or separated parents. The statistics are also very clear that a

> "Having a child with a disability is tough enough for a married couple, but is really difficult for a single parent."

child raised in a household with both parents is much more likely to be successful in school and in adult occupations (Nock, 1998). Children with a disability are no exception. It is logical that these children will need more help and support than those without disabilities. Having a child with a disability is tough enough for a married couple, but is really difficult for a single parent.

Two together are much better than one doing it alone. When one is down, or sick or away, the other person can pick up the slack. The ancient book of Ecclesiastes explains this in chapter 4 verses 9 - 12a [NLT]:

> Two people can accomplish more than twice as much as one;
>
> they get a better return for their labor. If one person falls,
>
> the other can reach out and help. But people who are alone
>
> when they fall are in real trouble. And on a cold night, two
>
> under the same blanket can gain warmth from each other.
>
> But how can one be warm alone? A person standing alone
>
> can be defeated, but two can stand back-to-back and conquer.

The consistent support for each other in a marriage is an absolute key to success for all members of the family.

We knew many single parents in our support group and all of them wished they could share the workload with another adult. It is not easy to get people to care for your child with a disability. Several of our single parents could not always make it to our once per month Monday night meetings because they could not find someone to watch their children for 2-3 hours. Many people are afraid they will do something wrong and shy away from taking responsibility for babysitting, providing transportation, or even helping with the other children in the family. However, everyone needs a break sometime. A single parent may find it nearly impossible to get a break unless it is from a family member or close friend. The impact on the child of a constantly stressed parent is not good.

Differences Between Husbands and Wives

I think we can all agree that women are not the same as men. This is true biologically for sure, but also in emotions, in temperament, in attitude, in relationship building, etc. If you want a little insight into the differences between you and your spouse, please grab two pieces of paper and each of you independently write down in rank order your top five needs in a marriage on the top half of the paper and what you think your spouse's top five needs in a marriage are on the bottom half of the paper. Single words or short phrases work fine. You should both end up with two lists ranked 1 to 5. No peeking until both of you are *completely* done.

Top Five Needs in a Marriage

My Needs:

1. _____

2. _____

3. _____

4. _____

5. _____

My Spouse's Needs:

1. _____

2. _____

3. _____

4. _____

5. _____

In a number of different groups, we have not seen two sets of lists that are generally close to each other. So, how did you do? Likely you were surprised by at least one or two things on your spouse's list and you wonder why some of the things on your list were not on his or her list (and the reverse also). Before you go any further, the parents need to eat out, go for a walk or out on a short drive and talk about your lists. Try to listen to why some of the things on your spouse's list of needs are there and why the items on your list for them were not there. Then reverse the discussion and explain why you selected and ordered your list of needs as you did. Do not be surprised if the wife's list is closer to the husband's list than the husband's list was for her. Women tend to be a little more insightful than men are about needs in marriage.

So how are you doing in meeting each other's needs? The gaps probably are a good place to start thinking about your marriage and your relationship. There is also likely to be a big difference in your needs as related to the children, especially the child with a disability. Fathers will tend to want to have measurable results and to see progress. Mothers tend to be relational and interested in how the child is feeling. One of the parents will tend to be more patient than the other parent about the rate of progress the child is making. This can be a major source of conflict and may be an area to work on together.

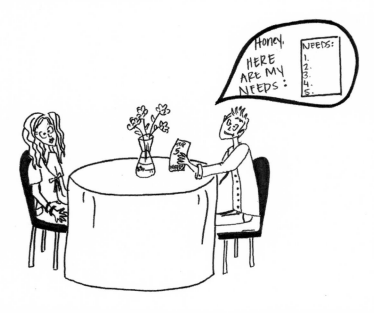

Actions and Reactions

While it is typical for a father to be less involved with the day-to-day raising of the children, he will also frequently set certain standards on what is acceptable behavior. The Bible and many contemporary advisors are full of advice on discipline and setting standards. The issue is not whether standards should be set, but rather *what* the standards should be and *how* they are set.

For argument's sake, say that the father sets pretty high standards such as minimum "B" grades in school, all chores done before dinner, children should always be respectful to each other and adults (especially family friends), etc. It is hard to argue that any of these are not desirable, but what if one or more of the children cannot achieve them? What if the child with the disability has poor social skills, does not know how to behave in front of adults, and cannot achieve the expected grades? The mother may develop more realistic standards and these will be in conflict with the father's standards. If the differences are not resolved, then conflict within the marriage will continue. The mother may start to make excuses for the child's behavior and may even start to keep secret much of their misbehavior from the father in order to protect them.

One last thought on actions and reactions that I have learned the slow and painful way is when a father is frustrated with his children and vents his frustrations to his wife—watch out! Mothers are typically more nurturing and emotionally closer to your children, so when you criticize the child, you are indirectly *criticizing the mother at the same time.* It took me years to realize this. I thought Gena was the one person I could safely vent my frustrations to. I discovered that discussing and complaining about almost anything *but the children* was relatively safe. My solution is to vent to friends about my issues with

> "Mothers are typically more nurturing and emotionally closer to your children, so when you criticize the child, you are indirectly criticizing the mother at the same time."

our children as much as possible. Be careful not to vent too much though so you do not lose your friend.

The Problem with Time

Another common problem is use of time. It is not unusual for the father to be the primary breadwinner and to feel that his primary role is to keep his job and work as hard at that as is possible. Therefore, the wife is very dependent on the husband for financial support and his time at home is limited. Many things around the home are usually best handled by the father such as fixing things, maintaining the property, maintaining the vehicles, etc. In addition, there may be things that the father and mother need to work on together such as cleaning windows (in our house for sure), driving the children around, etc.

It is also not unusual for the father to procrastinate on some of these jobs such as cleaning windows and fixing things. After all, he has a primary role of provider and may feel that he deserves time off from that. Only a few fathers will look at fixing or cleaning things as recreation or relaxation. Guess what the mother's reaction is to that leaky faucet that has not been fixed for a couple of weeks? Nagging! And this may be accompanied by reminders of all the other things she has asked him to do as well as the length of time it took him to finally do them.

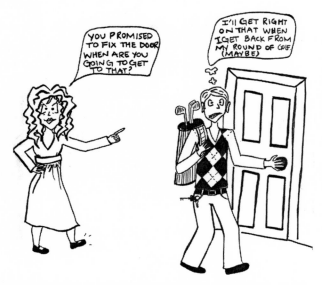

Parents of Children with Disabilities

There may be no getting around "time" issues in the marriage. We have struggled with these the entire 36 plus years of our marriage. Having a child with a disability frequently takes more time away from the marriage. Vacations are tough and sometimes almost impossible to manage. There was a time that I went to play golf at least once a week. We even joined a golf club for a few years and played together. It was fun, but it just took too much time. The only solution we have come up with is to openly discuss the time constraints and to try to come to a fair and formal resolution of what needs to be done and what free time each of you will be able to take. A lot of give and take may be needed, and do not expect to resolve this issue quickly. It will not stay static either as the family situation changes. The children get older, jobs change, friends change, and the family moves to a new city, etc. Adjustments to your fair and formal resolution will need to be made frequently. I would also emphasize the formal aspect of this discussion. Make sure each of you really understands what the other is expecting regarding the use of time. Writing down this understanding can be very helpful for accountability.

Another common problem is a lack of attentiveness and preoccupation by one of the parents. I have certainly tuned out the family at times. This usually happened when I was focused on work or focused on a project. When there are problems in the family, and especially when the problems are related to the child's disability, one of the parents might go into avoidance mode. It is a lot easier to avoid dealing with these difficult problems than to jump in with energy and focus. This was my approach at times I am sorry to have to admit. My priority was work or a project and not my family. I can remember building a very large deck that was almost the full width of the rear of our house and building it around a 15 x 30 foot above ground pool. I would come home from work at about 6:00 and jump into my work clothes and work until dark. Only then, dog tired, would I come in to spend time with the family. This put a heavy burden on Gena for many weeks. I justified it by saying the pool and deck were for the family; I was doing this all for the family. In reality, part of the reason was to avoid family issues and part of it was to accomplish something for myself. While the deck project was a success, we had to move shortly after that because I lost my job, and the project did not provide the benefits to the family I was sure it would.

Please be careful that you know your motives if you are really focused on work or projects or recreation and there is little time for the family. Could you be avoiding things? Is that business trip or socializing after work really necessary? Is spending hours on the computer or in front of the TV each day really necessary? I know of no parents who, when they looked back on their married life, wished they had spent *less* time with their families. We almost all wish we had spent more time with our spouse and with our children. The other things just take up time—valuable time. Who can remember the sitcom plot from your favorite show even two days later, the golf score last week, or the purpose of the business trip a few months ago?

> "I know of no parents who, when they looked back on their married life, wished they had spent less time with their families."

Strengthening the Marriage

Most of us are just too busy. If it is not work, then we fill our time with recreation or socializing. Marriages need to have undivided time to deal with the problems and issues that develop. Husbands and wives need to spend time alone together, without the children and without the daily grind. Children with special needs frequently require quality respite care people instead of teenage babysitters. This makes it more difficult for the couple to have time alone. We have not had any family living close to us since we got married. Our solution was the 30-hour getaway. We would drop our two children off at my mom's a 2 hour drive away and then spend Saturday into Sunday early afternoon going someplace, anyplace, twice a year. We went to Bed and Breakfast Inns and visited places all around the East Coast. We visited friends. It was not that important what we did, just that we spent time together. The time alone in the car to talk was helpful and so was the intimate time in a romantic location. If there is no fam-

> "If you have the ability, I highly recommend the 30-hour getaway!"

ily, consider trading off with friends. If you have the ability, I highly recommend the 30-hour getaway!

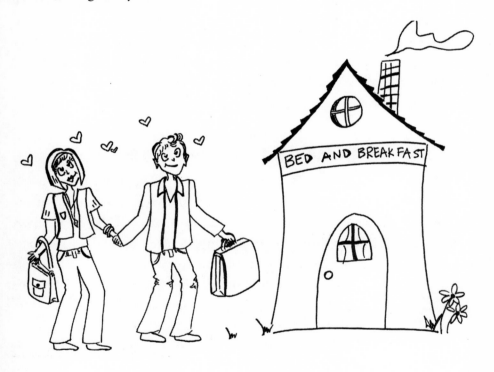

The second approach I recommend is to have each of you write down the 3 to 5 things that the other person could do to make the marriage better. Then compare notes at a time when you will not be interrupted for at least a few hours. A 30-hour getaway is a good time to do this. Be prepared to be surprised but also be prepared to exercise a lot of self control. Allow each other to talk uninterrupted for at least 10 minutes about each topic on their lists. Take turns with each person one item at a time. Do not expect to resolve things immediately. Let the ideas take time to develop. Change is not going to happen overnight.

The third approach I recommend is to attend a weekend marriage conference. We attended a "Marriage Encounter" weekend about 6-7 years into our marriage. It was a real benefit in helping us to gain a better understanding of each other. There was a lot of time alone and time to share ideas in a structured environment. We have since attended six marriage conferences over weekends. Each has been helpful in bringing out issues to talk over and in learning that our problems are not different from those faced by many other couples. Some of the innovative things other couples have done have been really interesting and helpful. Many of these conferences are Friday evening and all day Saturday formats.

Stay Married and Live Longer

There is a strong body of research that links increased longevity and better health with being married. According to a recent study, there is a clear relationship between marriage and longevity (Kaplan & Kronick, 2006). The report cites an average of an 18% increase in longevity for married couples. The report also indicated that marriage is very helpful in improving the longevity of the lives of the children. A spouse may help in catching ailments earlier and push a spouse and children to go to the doctor sooner and more often. A spouse provides a natural support mechanism to help deal with physical and emotional stress. Yes, even that hated nagging may actually help you live longer!

> "The report cites an average of an 18% increase in longevity for married couples."

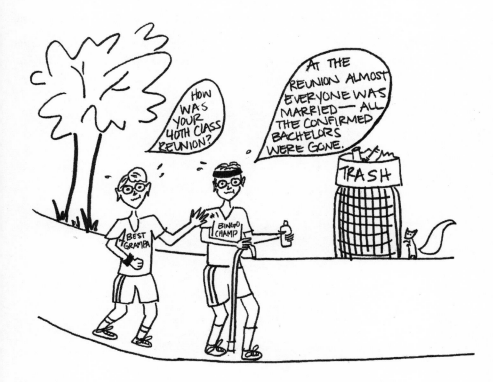

While living longer and healthier is obviously a good thing, there is also the issue of being there longer for your children – especially for your child with a disability. Who knows better how to help than you? If you are a significant supporter and advocate for your child, the longer you can do that the better it is for him or her. You may also be able to improve your financial position and therefore be better able to help your children when you are gone. Be sure to have a special needs trust set up if your child has received or will receive government support. Every state has a special needs trust provision. Without the special needs trust arrangement, the federal government has the right to be compensated for *all the expenses* they have incurred to help your child. This even includes the government's internal administration expenses!

This chapter just scratches the surface of marriage problems in families with disabilities. There are many very good resources on marriage that can help. One final thought – the marriage is precious in the eyes of God and is very important to the health and well-being of every member of the family. Make every effort to keep your marriage for yourselves, your family, and especially for your children.

Chapter Take-a-ways:

Work hard to improve your marriage.

Stay married if at all possible.

Live longer and healthier.

References

Kaplan, R. M., & Kronick, R. G. (2006). Marital status and longevity in the United States population. *Journal of Epidemiology & Community Health*, *60*(9), 760-765.

Nock, S. (1998). The family and hierarchy. *Journal of Marriage & Family*, *50*(4), 957- 966.

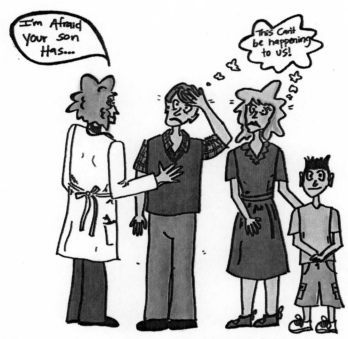

CHAPTER 6
Susan's Story

77

We were farmers, we were young, we were married, and we were really excited about our first child due any day. Kenton was 20 and I was 19 and everything was going great until 12 hours before Stephanie was born. My baby was in distress and the doctor was getting increasingly concerned. What was needed was a C-section, but he was not authorized to do it and did not call anyone in who could help. When Stephanie was born she was in extreme distress. She was not breathing and was having seizures. About 18 hours after birth she was life flighted to Children's Mercy Hospital where she stayed for the next 20 days.

The doctors then told us the sad news that our child would not be normal. Stephanie might be blind, but would very likely never walk and she had significant brain injury. They sent us home with lots of instructions and almost no support system and no training on how to take care of this tiny baby with so many challenges facing her and us.

I do not remember how we got through the first few months; it is just a blur from 29 years ago. I tried everything I could do to help her, but by the end of two months I was done. I hit a wall and could do no more. Stephanie was not blind but she had all sorts of physical problems and we were in the doctor's office a lot. I really tried to be Mrs. Fix it. I was not going to let this defeat me, but I just could not make Stephanie normal no matter how much I wanted to or tried. Kenton made his own attempt at being Mr. Fix it. He had the same results as my effort did, but it also put him into a period of depression. What he did do was to help me move more to acceptance of the situation instead of the constant fight to make it all better.

We fought the good fight for Stephanie for nine years as farmers but finally had to make the decision to leave farming and move to where there were better support systems. Stephanie had more and more medical problems the older she got. We were short of money all the time, felt uncertain of our future, and were under extreme stress. Kenton looks back at the early years and says that he, "kind of just had a hopeless feeling all the time." My dominant thought was that I was going to try to provide everything I could—no matter what.

In the city, Kenton got a full-time job with an elevator company but was laid off 4 ½ months later. I was forced to take a full-time job to get health benefits for the family. Kenton became Mr. Mom during the day and he worked part-time at night. Nine months later he was brought back and has been full-time ever since. We found a wonderful care provider that took care of Stephanie for 7 years and I was able to work during that time and improve our financial position.

Through most of this time I felt pretty stifled. Stephanie took up most of my time every day. We could take her out in the car but it was a major effort. Vacations were something that had to be meticulously planned out with lots of contingency plans if Stephanie had some type of medical emergency (which happened many times). There were numerous trips to the hospital emergency room when Stephanie had breathing problems. My life was centered on Stephanie. She was totally dependent on me and the family and we almost lost her quite a few times.

Family

I had a lot of support from our families and they had a lot of unconditional love for Stephanie. I was doing just what the doctors wanted me to do. We did the many surgeries and all the different therapies. My in-laws helped some but most of my family thought I was crazy doing all I did. We had two other wonder-

> "There is no doubt that Stephanie helped to mold their character into such wonderful people."

ful children that became more and more helpful as they grew older (and bigger than Stephanie). They learned how to do many therapies to help their older sister, to feed her, clean her, play with her, and to just love her. They also learned to be loving and caring people. There is no doubt that Stephanie helped to mold their character into such wonderful people. God truly can help all who believe in Him no matter what the circumstances.

Stephanie never got physically larger than the typical 7-year-old, even though she lived to adulthood. This was much longer than any doctor had said was possible. Only by the grace of God was she allowed this much time to be able to influence so many people in so many ways.

Faith

As a young couple we were not religious and did not really know God. I grew up as a Catholic and Kenton as a Presbyterian. I felt that I did not have a good faith model to follow. Kenton did, but the situation with Stephanie pulled him away from the church. So we left the church and put God on the back burner. We forgot Him, but He never forgot us. When Stephanie was 12 we felt there were spiritual needs in our lives that were not being met, especially for our children, so we started to go to a large Baptist church. We joined a small group and for the first time we felt truly loved and cared for. Unfortunately, the

> "We joined a small group and for the first time we felt truly loved and cared for."

love and care came from the small group and not from the church itself. The church never provided any real help despite our obvious need.

I was finally able to give my life to God and to put my children and our family in his care. This was really key when I was diagnosed with throat cancer. I survived the surgery and had a full recovery, but not without a major change in me and in our family. We realized the material things did not matter and Kenton stopped taking overtime and out-of-town trips to make extra money. God had used this trying and scary time to change us and change us for the better. Our church and our small group helped all of us come to a saving relationship with Christ.

The Later Years

Until age 21, Stephanie was able to get a lot of help from the school system. At age 21 she graduated and I had a huge cry. All that support was suddenly gone! It took us 1 ½ years to get the state to finally provide some services 2 days a week for a total of 10 hours per week. I felt those 18 months had really moved us backwards. But God blessed us with a wonderful couple that took Stephanie bowling, roller skating, swimming, and to the theater. However, because of our increased financial needs, Kenton started to work longer hours and I felt I was alone again. This was a most difficult time for our marriage and our family.

Finally we found an organization that was focused on helping adults with severe disabilities. They had a center very close to where I worked and they helped develop Stephanie's skills. I was now able to leave Stephanie there for up to 30 hours per week. What a blessing this was. She received excellent care and therapy. At times, Stephanie was allowed to come to work with me. Again, this was a great blessing. I do not think many organizations welcome children to the workplace!

A few years earlier we had to make a decision about a feeding tube. It was getting harder and harder to feed Stephanie and was almost a battle to get nourishment into her. She was not getting enough nourishment from her special diet because she had trouble swallowing and keeping the food down. We are not quick decision makers and we prayed and agonized over this for months. The issue was really our issue, not Stephanie's. For me, the feeding sessions were one of the last normal activities we had with Stephanie. Giving this up was like admitting failure. We finally did have the feeding tube put in and Stephanie quickly got much healthier.

Other's Point of View

One of the big problems we had was the lack of understanding by other people and families. Stephanie was very disabled. She could not walk or talk, was tiny for her age, and generally not very responsive to others. People did

> "People did not know how to react to her and the natural tendency for them was to avoid us."

not know how to react to her and the natural tendency for them was to avoid us. Gradually this changed as people came to know us, but it was hard to say the least. We frequently had little children ask, "What's wrong with her?" We had no problem answering, but the parents were generally upset by the questions from their children. Our friends were very accepting and we found we could take Stephanie out with us to church events and family events with little difficulty. Stephanie really liked to get out and do things.

What We Learned

One of the most important lessons we learned is that we are not in charge. Both Kenton and I are the kind of people that want order in our lives and want to have a measure of control over things. What happened to Stephanie was a tragedy without a doubt. But it led to so many wonderful opportunities. Our two other children grew up in a family that needed to stick together and work together. They became very compassionate and responsible people because of this. I became an outward focused person instead of an inward focused person.

We determined very early that our other two children deserved special attention as much as Stephanie did. We made an effort on a regular basis to do something special with each of them. Kenton made a point of taking each of our other two children out to dinner on a regular basis and we had special birthday parties for each of them. We went on a family vacation every year from the time our youngest was age 5.

"The trouble with grieving over a child with a permanent disability is that the grief has no real end."

Grieving was difficult—especially in the first 2 years. I kept asking myself, why me? Why did this have to happen? The trouble with grieving over a child with a permanent disability is that the grief has no real end. For most people facing a tragedy, there is the tragic event followed by a period of grief and healing. With my type of situation the grief goes on as each day has the same sense of loss as the day before and the day to come. What made all the difference to me was having God take control. He is in charge. My grief pushed me into a life saving relationship with Jesus. Without Stephanie, that might not have happened. The same is true for our entire family.

We spent a lot of time with doctors and therapists and all different kinds of care givers and bureaucrats. We learned to be patient and to seek out the ones that really cared as opposed to those that just wanted to do their job. Doctors usually cared, but we found we had to take what they said with a grain of salt. They have a tendency to think they always know what is best. This is not true. As parents we knew our daughter better than any of the doctors ever would. So we made decisions that were not always in agreement with the doctors. Looking back over the 27 years, I can honestly say that we do not regret any of the decisions we made. We took our time, we studied, we prayed, and we decided.

A tragedy can really have an impact on a marriage. With Kenton and I, it was really challenging in the early years and then again when Stephanie lost the school system support. But the great thing is that it forced us together more than it forced us apart. We stood together in dealing with our family, in dealing with the doctors and the emergencies, in dealing with the bureaucracies, and in dealing with the impact of the outside world on our family. We are stronger now than we ever would have been without Stephanie!

Stephanie changed so many lives. At the place I worked, many people grew to love Stephanie, and I realized what a positive impact she had on many people with all sorts of issues of their own. I remember the day a lady with a child with a disability met me and Stephanie. She was a relatively new mother and was very distraught about her child's condition. She asked me, "How do you do it?" I just smiled and said, "You just love them." She thought about this for a minute as she looked at us and then put up a great big smile and said, "OK, I can do this!"

> "We are stronger now than we ever would have been without Stephanie!"

Conclusion

One Sunday morning in the winter of 2007, Stephanie unexpectedly passed away. She is with the Lord with a new body and a new life. We grieve for the loss of our daughter, but delight in her life in heaven. She changed everything for us and many others and we are much better people for knowing her.

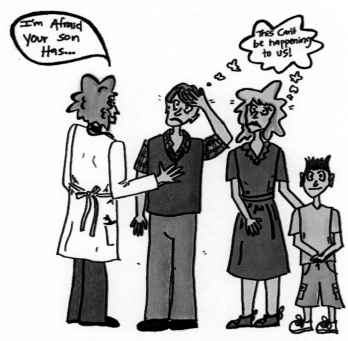

CHAPTER 7
Friendships

87

J oshua and Ruth were a well-liked couple with many friends in their neighborhood and friends they had kept from college and even from high school. They had two children: Drew, age 10, and Morgan, age 7. The family lived in a rural area and the closest major city was about 60 miles away. Morgan was a real tomboy and loved to climb the trees in their back yard. Last year she was climbing in the trees when a quick rain shower popped up. As she was climbing down she slipped and fell the last 8 feet. Unfortunately, she fell on her back. She felt a lot of pain and Ruth heard her screaming from the house. With some difficulty in the rain, Ruth got her into the car and they rushed over to the doctor's office in the town 9 miles away. The doctor quickly decided that Morgan needed to go to the hospital. She was given a shot for the pain, strapped on a gurney and rushed to the city hospital.

One year later, Morgan still cannot walk, as there was severe damage to her lower spine. Despite two surgeries and many months of physical therapy, she uses a wheel chair. With a lot of support, she can walk a few paces and is able to use the bathroom with minimal assistance. She is able to go to school on a special bus, but needs help to get on and off the bus. The doctors are optimistic that Morgan will be able to walk some day if she continues with the physical therapy on a regular basis and has one more surgery when she has finished her adolescent growth period in a few years. Therapy is only available in the city and the 2-hour round trip is expensive and takes a lot of time and money. Insurance is starting to be a problem as the costs have reached over $200,000 with no end in sight. Joshua's employer has started to ask about Morgan a lot and they seem to be very concerned with the increased insurance premiums the firm is paying. Joshua and Ruth have started to talk about moving to the city to be nearer the physical therapists, the specialists, and the hospital if Morgan continues to have back spasms.

As they look back at last year, they see changes in their social lives. Morgan's best friend Tammy has stopped visiting all together and Morgan says she feels like she is being left out of many social things at school. Ruth's best friend Mary has been wonderful and they have grown even closer to each other. Tom and Carol have also become good friends. Their son has autism and both couples have found it helpful to meet in each other's homes a couple of times each month. Ruth has lost a number of friends she used to shop and have lunch with just because she does not have the free time she used to have. A few friends at church with children the same age as Morgan have slipped away. Joshua cut back on going to the Elks club so he can help Ruth with Morgan when he gets home from work. Their home feels a little more isolated than it used to. The co-pay on the medical insurance has really cut into their finances and they skipped their usual trip to Ruth's family this year as it was too costly. The 6-hour drive is also too difficult for Morgan despite the used handicapped accessible van they purchased.

Friendships are hard to find and can be harder to keep when life brings major challenges to a family. These are some of the keys to developing and keeping friends:

1. Be committed to each other and do not let events drive you apart.

2. Share confidences with each other.

3. Be there unconditionally for each other.

4. Share and celebrate each other's achievements.

5. Bring fun and joy into each other's lives.

6. Make the time to get together and to communicate on a regular basis.

7. Cherish the past, present, and future times in the relationship.

As we see from the story of Joshua and Ruth, a child with a disability can have a profound impact on friendships both before and after the disability. As we read above, some of the friends allowed the event to create problems with the friendships. Some people do not know how to deal with disabilities. They may feel awkward around the child and not know what to say for fear of saying the wrong thing. The other children may shy away from them, especially if they can no longer play as they used to or if the disability prevents communication and is scary to the other children. This can lead the parents to also shy away from the family.

Because the disability will likely require the parents to change their time and energy commitments, friends that needed a lot of time and energy may easily fall away. Commitments to things like baseball teams or bridge clubs may become too time-consuming to continue and the friends made while attending those activities may fall away. The lack of a common interest will strain many relationships. If the child with a disability needs continual and daily support, then the time for friends can be very limited. As in the story above, Ruth could not leave Morgan for any extended time. Children with a severe illness or developmental disability typically require a trained care provider. Susan's story (Chapter 6) is a great example of how time consuming this can be. It can be pretty hard to meet friends in places like doctor's offices and physical therapy centers.

Gena and I have had problems with our lack of available time for friends for many decades. Part of this has been the time needed to be there for our son. Some vacations and events did not happen because of our inability to find suitable coverage. The provision of a qualified person to care for a child with a disability is called respite care. There is a severe shortage of people that can and are willing to care for a child with disabilities. For many parents, the major source of respite care will be family. A trusted family member that is able and willing to provide respite care is a great benefit. Every parent needs some respite from the day in and day out care giving.

Parents need someone they can relate to and can share their feelings with. As discussed earlier, most men generally have no one they can share with. Fathers of a child with a disability need to find someone they can talk to about their situation. Likewise, mothers have the same need – only more so if they are the primary care provider for the child. A friend that a parent can talk to in confidence is very important. Joshua and Ruth found another couple in a similar situation and they became good friends. Your changed situation may lead to different friends, and maybe even to better and deeper friendships.

> "Your changed situation may lead to different friends, and maybe even to better and deeper friendships."

Single Parents

All of these difficulties are even more profound for the single parent. The time constraints are usually much more difficult as there is no one to share the burdens. Finances are frequently more strained with only one person to provide income for the family and child support payments are not always reliable. Strains with the previous other parent and their family can add to the emotional burden.

A few suggestions that we have gathered from single parents are that first being close to family is a big help. Grandparents can frequently be very helpful and they are tied into the family and usually care about their child and grandchildren. A brother or sister in the area can also be a great help. A good second choice is to have a good reliable friend or two. In the absence of family, they can fill this role. Furthermore, a church or Bible study group can be a great help. Many single parents told us that their church had made a real difference in providing some respite care and emotional support.

Another suggestion is to join a support group. Many support groups are created by single caregivers seeking support and guidance. The major advantage these groups have is the depth of understanding of the challenges facing the single caregiver. Unfortunately, many of them are also burdened by time and financial issues. A key way single caregivers can support each other is to have time when one person watches their own children along with the children of other parents. This gives each parent some free time, which is a precious commodity. Financially, the sharing of the children can also save on expenses. The parent watching the other children can receive some compensation and usually this benefits the other parents as it is a lot cheaper than paying a certified child-care worker. Lastly, some single parents have found friends and support on the Internet. Not only is this a great place to gather information but you can meet in social group forums and swap ideas and stories.

Changed Lifestyle

For many families, there may be a need for changes in the family's lifestyle. Financial issues can dominate if medical insurance is poor or not available. Employers may terminate employment if costs become too high. As the story above discusses, there may be a need to relocate to support the child with a disability. We have seen many cases where the family relocated to a different school district or even to a different state to obtain needed educational and medical supports for their child. Better benefits are frequently found in governmental jobs or with large firms. International firms seem to be somewhat better than U.S. firms, as they come from an environment where medical care is a given for all people. Finding new friends is a challenge in a new location for anyone. Those families who have a child with special needs might find it more challenging as you will be limited to where you can meet new people. We have found that the local church can be a great source of support and a place to meet friends. Two of our very best couple friends are people we met in Bible studies. We also met Susan (see Susan's story) in a small Bible study group.

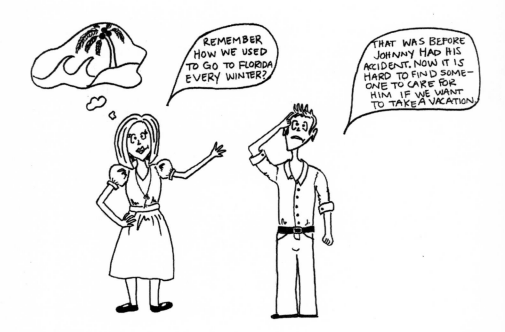

One of the keys to developing friendships is to be willing to open up to people and to share confidences. Susan and her husband Kenton were open with the group and therefore we were able to help them where and when they needed help. Likewise, we were also open with our small group and they were able to help us because they knew what our needs were. Opening up to others is not easy for many people. We believe that there is sometimes a sense of shame in the family, and to some extent, there may also be some embarrassment. Unfortunately, many parents feel that their child's disability reflects on them in some way. We found this to be true with developmental disabilities such as au-

> "Unfortunately, many parents feel that their child's disability reflects on them in some way."

tism and Asperger Syndrome. This reflection on the parents may have been due to old but inaccurate ideas that the conditions were due to bad parenting and inherited genetic properties.

There is also the issue that the parent should have been able to protect the child somehow, and many parents have this lingering guilt. All of this adds to the difficulty in talking about the situation with others. A support group for parents with similar problems is a safer place to open up to others. We highly recommend that you actively look to meet other families dealing with similar disabilities. We found that opening up to others not only helped us but we were able to help them. If you want to feel better yourself, there is no better way than to help someone who is in real need.

It is important to remember that your child is not just your child, but also God's child. We believe that God loves and values all of his children. Jesus made it very clear to his disciples that he loved them and considered them his friends. In John 15:14 Jesus calls his disciples friends because he taught them all they needed to know about the Father. We have the same opportunity to learn about God through the guidance of the scriptures and the Holy Spirit. Jesus is our friend. He is a friend that will never leave us, never forget us and will always be there to help us. A believer in Jesus is never alone. Jesus clearly stated that he especially loved children. One time when Jesus was speaking, some children were brought to him, but

> **"Jesus is our friend. He is a friend that will never leave us, never forget us and will always be there to help us."**

the disciples rebuked the parents for distracting Him. In Matthew 19:14 (NIV) Jesus said, "Let the little children come to me, and do not hinder them, for the kingdom of heaven belongs to such as these." There is every reason to believe that Jesus loves all children, those with or without a disability.

Interestingly, God's church is not always the best place to find support. Some church leaders view people with disabilities as distractions. A previous pastor refused to provide any worship accommodations for several individuals with disabilities because he apparently felt they would be distracting during the worship service. The church had adults with cerebral palsy stay in the back of the worship center because their involuntary arm movements and noises were distracting. We tried for years to have this large church provide an area in the worship center for those with disabilities, but were not successful. Interestingly, the church eventually did provide signing for the deaf in the front of the worship center. In the city where we live now, we are only aware of a few churches that actively accommodate people with disabilities in their worship services. We personally doubt very much that Jesus would want His church to discourage people with disabilities from attending worship services.

Your spouse should be your greatest confidant. You need to trust your spouse with many fears, concerns, and worries that you know will not be passed on to any other person. This requires that each of you have real trust in each other. A good friend is also someone you can talk to and trust. Just as in marriage, this takes time and effort. Maybe you are very blessed and have a friend or two you have known for years that you can talk to. Many do not have such a friend and really need friends. As I discussed earlier, I found myself in this situation about ten years ago. I made a decision to start a men's group with some men from our neighborhood and our church. It took a year or two, but I had some friends that I could share my problems and worries with in complete trust.

We clearly should share in the successes and achievements of our spouses and our friends. This is a great way to show that we care. They are very likely to return the favor and support you in your successes and achievements. This needs to go beyond just celebrating birthdays and giving presents on holidays. The first love language, words of affirmation, is the key. You need to do just the opposite of what Archie Bunker did on the comedy show *All In The Family*. Archie explained to Edith (his wife) that he told her he loved her when they got married, and he would let her know if he changed his mind. Spouses and friends are not mind readers and they need to be (and deserve to be) reminded of how much you care for them. For more information on the languages of love, see Gary Chapman's book entitled, *The Five Love Languages: How to Express Heartfelt Commitment to Your Mate.*

> "You need to do just the opposite of what Archie Bunker did on the comedy show *All In The Family.* Archie explained to Edith (his wife) that he told her he loved her when they got married, and he would let her know if he changed his mind."

Obstacles to Friendships

We have already talked about the time problem. Lack of time is a well-documented problem for most Americans. Americans work more hours in the average year than workers in most western nations and get less vacation and time off. Taking care of a person with a disability also takes energy. Many people we know in this situation are just too tired. I ran into a woman recently who had a child with severe allergic reactions during her entire childhood. She indicated to me that she was just so tired from helping her child that she had no real energy or time left for herself and for developing friendships. Many primary care providers essentially put their social lives on hold because of a lack of time and energy. As discussed earlier, this can lead to feelings of loneliness and can lead to depression. One parent recently remarked to me, "I just do not feel I can do more than just keep going." Taking care of one's basic needs and being the primary care giver for another is about all many of us can handle. This parent went on to say that she felt isolated from others and was convinced that there was no easy way to reconnect for her.

We usually meet new people at activities or through other friends. If you are already lacking in friends, then you may be limited to meeting people at activities. These activities frequently require you to find someone to watch your child while you attend the event. For young children, this might mean a family member or a well-qualified teenager. For older children or children with moderate or severe disabilities, it may require a qualified respite care provider. There is a real shortage of these people in most places. Perhaps a local university or college would have a training program for respite care providers to help reduce the shortage.

Sometimes government programs will provide some money for respite care. In Missouri, this was limited to $500 per year for persons with developmental disabilities. In other states, it may not be not provided at all. Respite care is also needed by the parents just to have some time for each other. At least one week every year or two devoted to nourishing the marriage is what we found most parents needed. The cost of respite care can more than double the cost of a vacation and can easily consume your entire year's respite allowance money.

God's clear priority is for family. It is written in I Timothy 5:8 (NIV), "If anyone does not provide for his relatives, and especially for his immediate family, he has denied the faith and is worse than an unbeliever." We are in a situation where we have to make choices about where we put our time, energy, and focus. If God has put a person with a disability in your life to care for, then it is likely this is a top priority he has assigned to you. Friends are needed, but family will likely have to come first. God has promised a reward for those who are obedient to his commands. As you take care of your family, you are doing God's will.

> "If God has put a person with a disability in your life to care for, then it is likely this is a top priority he has assigned to you."

There is no easy method for developing and maintaining friendships. If there is a support group in your area, I would encourage you to go. You will likely learn some interesting and relevant information about the disability you are dealing with. More importantly, you will have a chance to meet people like yourselves. If you are older, then helping younger parents can be very rewarding. If you are newly involved with your situation, make an effort to seek out those that are more experienced. We felt that a support group was needed in our area, and made the decision to start one. If there is no group you can find, you, too, can make an effort to start one.

Experts from local colleges and universities as well as government organizations can be a source of information and support. Many faculty members in higher education have community outreach as part of their goals and objectives. The special education faculty would be a prime group to contact. Your school district might also be willing to sponsor or support you. The schools know which children are in special education classes and can help you find families that might be interested in a support group. If you have a child receiving special education from the school system, then increasing your visibility with the special education leadership may help you in getting the services you need for your child. In fact, every member of your support group can gain this benefit if they are actively involved.

Chapter Take-a-ways:

Having friends is worth the time and effort.

Work to make your spouse your best friend.

Family has to be the top priority.

Jesus is your friend no matter the circumstances.

References

Chapman, G. (1995). *The five love languages: How to express heartfelt commitment to your mate.* Chicago: Moody Press.

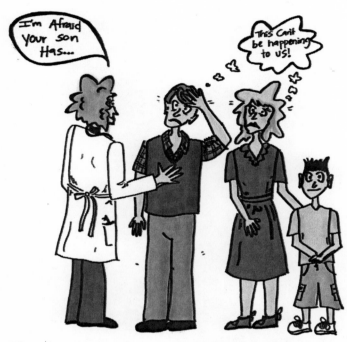

CHAPTER 8
Discipline

101

D iscipline in our home has never been easy. The first problem we had was that discipline was very different between our two sets of parents. Gena's family tended to be louder and punishment oriented. My family was more reserved and used threats of consequences to control behavior. Gena had two younger brothers and I had two younger sisters. Each of us had only one family to learn from, and being first-born children meant our parents were still learning how to parent when we were growing up. Expectations were higher for us than our younger siblings and discipline was firm. This pattern is typical. As parents get more experienced, they frequently become more flexible. Flexibility and consistency are the keys to proper discipline in a family with a child with disabilities.

Disciplining a child with special needs can be a challenge in terms of fairness, type of discipline, and impact on relationships. Discipline is needed to teach and guide behavior, to enforce natural consequences, and to build character. *The Oxford American College Dictionary* defines discipline as "the practice of training people to obey the rules or a code of behavior, using punishment to correct disobedience" (p. 387). Furthermore, the definition of disciplining oneself to do something is to "train oneself to do something in a controlled and habitual way" (p. 387). Unfortunately, discipline is frequently used by some parents to force a child to do one's wishes. Also, the punishment aspect is focused on more than the training and teaching. Punishment may get you what you want at the moment, but you may not want what you get in the long-term.

This is because using punishment alone as a consequence can produce many unintended effects such as resentment. Parents need to know what they are doing if they want to have a positive impact! Training and teaching is needed; however, it sure can be misapplied.

Phillip always had trouble controlling his temper. Now that he is married to June and they have three children, there are plenty of times he feels he is losing his cool and lashing out. Their son Keith is now 12 and has Down syndrome. Keith is able to function well as long as everyone is patient and able to make sure he understands exactly what he is supposed to do and he is given reminders as needed. Just last week, Keith got mad at dinner and threw his plate of food on the floor. June knew that Keith had not been feeling well but forgot to tell Phillip before dinner. Phillip verbally unloaded on Keith, and Keith started crying and curled up into a ball in the hallway. Needless to say, dinner was ruined for everyone. Phillip felt pretty bad after he had a chance to cool down and June felt bad because she had not talked to Phillip before dinner. They worked together to get Keith calmed down and finally to bed. Keith avoided his dad for the next few weeks, as he was afraid of another verbal assault. He also did poorly at school and he tried to avoid eating with Phillip.

Phillip and June's daughter Lisa, age 9, and son Tommy, age 7, are both doing fine but are starting to resent the fact that Keith is allowed to get away with things that they are punished for or are not allowed to do. A rule that Phillip has in his house is that all homework needs to be finished before the children can watch TV on weekdays and Sunday nights before school. While Keith has only a little homework to do, there are times he cannot calm down enough to work on it. His disability prevents him from having the concentration he needs. Many times if he has had a bad day at school, an hour of TV can take his mind off the day's events and allow him to do his homework in the evening. Last Wednesday June caught Lisa watching TV with Keith right after school. She had obviously broken the TV rule. She was punished with no TV that evening and on Thursday night when her favorite show was airing. She threw a fit, screaming, "This is not fair! How come Keith watches TV after school and I can't?"

First, you need to decide what the goal of discipline is. Do you just want obedience or do you want the child to develop his or her character? Do you want your child to fear you or to love you? Next, you need to determine what is appropriate for your child with a disability and for your other children. Sometimes the same disciplinary approach such as implementing time-outs or losing a privilege or desired activity can work for both. However, you may have to develop a special set of options for your child with a disability. Discipline is not the same as punishment. In fact, punishment can produce many unintended effects such as building resentment. Discipline should teach the appropriate behavior expected as well as provide consequences for misbehavior.

Children with severe disabilities may have so much pain and difficulty in their life that some forms of punishment and discipline may be unfair. Your other children may have to be disciplined completely differently and will need to understand why their sibling is not being treated in the same way. For psychological and emotional disabilities, this can be especially hard because the other children might not be able to understand the reasons that justify the different type or intensity of discipline. You also need to consider that there may be a significant difference between the chronological age of a child and his or her emotional age. A 13-year-old whose emotional

> "Your other children may have to be disciplined completely differently and will need to understand why their sibling is not being treated in the same way."

functioning is similar to a typical 6-year-old will not understand the logic that other 13-year-olds do and therefore cannot be expected to behave like a typical 13-year-old. You will need to spend time explaining to your other children why consequences are different for the sibling with a disability. Do not expect full acceptance of this two-tiered approach from the other children. If you are consistent with your approach, they will come to accept the situation. Of course, your teaching approaches will change as the children change and grow older, too.

The lenient approach was very popular back in the 1960s. This was very unfair to the children. Parents need to mold the values of their children. Withholding discipline in a sense just allows the child to self-select their values. If the parents are not active in this process then the children will get most of their values from their peers. Children learning values from other children is *not* a recipe for success!

Team Discipline

It is critical that you and your spouse are "on the same page" in terms of how you approach discipline and how you define your goals. The only way to be totally in harmony is to agree ahead of time how to handle each situation. It is impossible to predict these situations so your only recourse is to agree on a set of guidelines. These will vary greatly from family to family. The important action is to regularly review your situation together, make appropriate adjustments and firmly agree on your approach. Your failure in this area will lead to the child playing favorites with the more lenient parent, and this will be a wedge between you and your spouse.

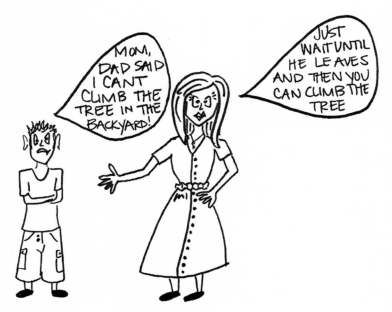

Consistency is a key to fair and effective discipline. Failure to do chores or schoolwork or therapy needs to have a consistent consequence. Being inconsistent will confuse the child and could easily lead to inconsistent behavior as the child tests to see what he or she can get away with. The other children will also notice any inconsistency and their behavior may also lead to testing your limits. The consistency needs to be between the parents and also from each parent. Each parent must apply the rules and consequences fairly and uniformly. Letting the child get away with something just once can lead to efforts to beg for mercy every time a consequence is being applied.

A solid approach is actually creating natural consequences for the child's behavior. The best way to put this into practice is to have a written agreement within the family of what is expected and what happens if things do not happen that way. It becomes a natural consequence instead of punitive. If your son fails to clean up his room, he lives in a messy room and probably loses many of his things. Consistently applied, the conse-

> "Being inconsistent will confuse the child and could easily lead to inconsistent behavior as the child tests to see what he or she can get away with."

quences can even become automatic and the child accepts the consequence as a natural and expected event. For small children, pictures on the refrigerator can provide a visual support of natural consequences.

For older children and even adults, a written contract signed by both the parents and the child may be appropriate. Brent actually asked us to do this when he was 22, and the consequences that he recommended were harsher than we would have suggested. Gena worked with him to make the consequences more reasonable. When it came time to implement the consequence because Brent failed to do what he had promised in his contract, he said that he lost the contract he wrote. He was quite shocked when Gena retrieved the Xerox copy she had made of it and presented it to him. Brent's sense of time was short and he had a difficult time relating future consequences to his feelings and behavior at the moment.

Consequences need to be immediate so the child can understand the relationship between the behavior and the consequence. Our daughter did not like this either, as it forced her to be accountable for her actions and because she could see how poorly Brent did. However, this approach does give the child a sense of control. It also helps children develop their character in the area of responsibility and in understanding that there are consequences to making mistakes. A great positive of this approach is that when the behavioral goals are met, there are positive rewards for both the child and for the family. For example, a trip to the ice cream store could happen every week that there are positive results.

Discipline is hard work. It should be done in love and never in anger. This is a lot easier said than done. The old adage of counting to 10 before you discipline or react is good advice. There were times when we were not in good emotional control when disciplining our children. Obviously, the discipline needs to be appropriate to the situation and just to repeat one more time, both you and your spouse need to be on the same page as to what is appropriate.

Like Father Like Son?
Like Mother Like Daughter?

You are very likely to be disciplining your children pretty much the way your parents disciplined you. Most of us have not had any formal training on discipline. However, fair discipline for the child with special needs may be very different than the discipline you experienced as a child. It is right and proper to be unbalanced with your discipline in this situation. What seemed to work for your parents may not be appropriate for you in your situation. You may have to change; you may need help to develop a two-tiered discipline approach for your family. Your spouse, professionals, other parents with children with disabilities like yours, or other trusted parents are the ones to help you with this.

The single parent may have their own set of issues with discipline. Obviously they are the only disciplinarian at home since the spouse is not there to share the load. Secondly, the single parent has only his or her set of experiences to draw upon in making discipline decisions. Sometimes they are good and appropriate experiences and sometimes they are not. When things are out of control, it is just you and the children. No one is there to discuss what went wrong. On the positive side, at least no one is there second guessing things!

The Bible is full of great advice on disciplining children. The very first verses of the first chapter of Proverbs discuss attaining wisdom and discipline. Later in Proverbs 23:13a (NIV) we read, "Do not withhold discipline from a child," and in Proverbs 29:17(NIV), "Discipline your son, and he will give you peace; he will bring delight to your soul." We all need to be disciplined to correct our mistakes and to learn right from wrong. Withholding discipline is foolish as it deprives the child of the ability to grow and to learn from his or her mistakes. Discipline shows love and passes on your values to your children. You will discipline your children if you love them and want what is best for them. You only discipline if you care. Try to never discipline in anger, and only discipline to help the child learn from his or her mistakes. Failure to discipline only shows that the parent is unwilling to do what is hard and necessary. It takes work and effort to discipline fairly and consistently. Shirking that duty is wrong, and is avoiding a prime responsibility of parenting. Disciplining is synonymous with teaching.

Over disciplining is just as bad as too little discipline. As Colossians 3:21 (NIV) says, "Fathers, do not embitter your children, or they will become discouraged." We may try strict discipline and many rules to try to gain control over what seems to be an uncontrollable situation. Children need discipline, but you can embitter your children by trying to be over controlling or by using them to do your disciplining for you. For example, a family with a child with bi-polar disorder may have many days when the child is manic and very hard to keep quiet and on task. If there are strict rules that *all* the children have to be done with their chores and homework before TV and the child with the disorder is not done, it may be unfair to apply the consequences to everyone. Having the

> **"If you find yourself making more and more rules to try to gain control in the family, be careful."**

other children put pressure on the child with special needs to conform to the rules can also be counterproductive and lead to resentment. This may work at times, but *you* are the parent and discipline is *your* responsibility, not theirs.

Being too strict is a great way to make everyone unhappy. Your other children will become resentful of your rules and will likely be resentful of their sibling with special needs, too. If you find yourself making more and more rules to try to gain control in the family, be careful. Talk it over with your spouse and be prepared to give up some control. Use all means to have full agreement between you and your spouse on consequences and punishment for behavior. If you are single, talk to a friend, other family member, or a trained counselor.

How Do You and Your Spouse View Discipline?

The reason we have included a chapter on discipline is not just because it is so difficult in families who have a child with special needs, but rather because discipline is also a great source of conflict between the parents. Each parent may have a different approach and a different attitude about discipline. There is a large body of research showing that positive reinforcement is what works best. This approach may be acceptable to one parent, but not to the other parent. Many parents grew up in homes where negative consequences were applied for misbehavior. When one of the children did something wrong they were punished. There may have been few, if any, rewards for good behavior. In simple terms, children were to follow the rules and were punished when they did not follow the rules. All children were subject to the same rules. However, punishment alone does not teach the children how to act appropriately and one of the purposes of discipline is to teach. Children must be taught how to perform the expected behaviors. We cannot assume that they know how to do this without instruction.

In your situation, all children being subject to the same "fair" rules probably will not work. Nevertheless, that may be what you learned from your parents and it may seem fair and balanced. Each of us only gets one family to learn from and to grow up in. For many of us, the approach used by our parents seems like the right way. We survived and it worked, or at least seemed to work. We may have to go through an unlearn-

> "Fair does not mean equal. It means providing each child with what he or she needs. In a sense, we are leveling the playing field for the child with a disability."

ing phase before we can learn a new way. If the parents come from very different backgrounds, these differences can be hard to reconcile. Fair does not mean equal. It means providing each child with what he or she needs. In a sense, we are leveling the playing field for the child with a disability.

My family almost never used physical punishment. Angry words were also fairly rare. My father was very focused on his work and left running the home to my mother. I had two younger sisters and they were very good at manipulating situations to their advantage. My mother was an only child herself, so she had no experience with siblings. A common solution to an argument was to take a vote. Guess who was out voted almost every time? I learned to spend a lot of time in my room with the door locked. If I had done something "really bad," my mother would have my father deal with it when he got home. Gena's family was very different. Her father was dealing with alcoholism, and worked long hours at a job with a 2-hour commute each way. Her mother was the primary disciplinarian because her husband was away so much and was not in good self-control when he came home.

We came from families with different approaches to punishment and discipline. It took a lot of hard work to reconcile our thoughts on discipline and punishment. We were very unprepared for the issues of discipline for a child with special needs. As we discuss in other parts of the book, I was really in denial that Brent was disabled. I therefore held him to behavior standards that he really could not meet. This was unfair to Brent and was a serious challenge in our marriage. As with many disabilities, it can be very difficult to determine the behavior level at which to hold the child accountable. Gena knew Brent much better than I did and I eventually let her guide our discipline approaches with Brent.

Discipline in the family can become a power struggle between the spouses if there are significant differences of opinion. This can also be a control issue for the spouses. The family background may be a factor in terms of which parent was the disciplinarian in the two families. Most of us need to really understand and review what we learned about discipline when we were growing up. Your parents were probably at least as inexperienced as you are! They made mistakes that may have been passed down the generations on both sides of the family. There are a large number of books and other resources on discipline and I would urge you to take a look at a few of these together. Talk to other families in situations similar to yours.

In summary, discipline is a difficult but very important function that is needed to help children grow, to know right from wrong, and to develop the proper values. Discipline is a very difficult task for parents of a child with special needs. You will need to devote a lot of time and effort to get it right.

Chapter Take-a-ways:

Discipline is essential for all children.

Discipline requires training to do it right.

Discipline is fair if it is relative to the child's abilities.

Be consistent and under control when disciplining.

Make sure that both spouses are on the same page.

References

Lindberg, C. A. (2002). *The Oxford American college dictionary.* New York: Oxford University Press.

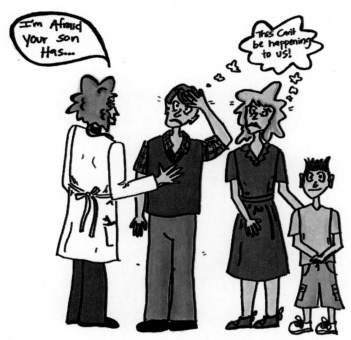

CHAPTER 9
How to Help Yourself

115

I t will be a rare parent that is not blown away by the situation you find yourself in. Few of us are really prepared to handle a family, let alone a child with a disability in the family. Let me make one thing clear at the start: If you are not able to function well, then you will be unable to do much to help your family. You owe it to yourself and to your family to get better. This is a fight you need to keep fighting and you cannot afford to lose.

Shawn and Darcy are a middle thirties couple and their second child, a girl, was born last year with cystic fibrosis. It was a tremendous shock as their first daughter who is now 4 is growing up normally with none of her sister's problems. After the first shock and the first months when it seemed she was in the hospital constantly, things have settled down some and her prognosis for the near term is not too bad.

Their pastor recommended a support group for children with disabilities held at a neighboring church and this has been a great help. Shawn and Darcy have met with families that have similar problems and learned some of the ways they have adjusted. They joined the National Cystic Fibrosis Foundation and learned a lot about the disease, treatments, and ways to cope with the pressures and worries. They feel a little better being equipped with this knowledge but still feel down about the future.

The good news is that neither Shawn nor Darcy nor you have to fight this fight alone. There are millions of parents fighting these fights, and there are many people and many organizations that are willing and able to help you. You would not be reading this book if you were content with your situation. Reading a book is one of the many ways you can help yourself. First, you need to gain insight about yourself.

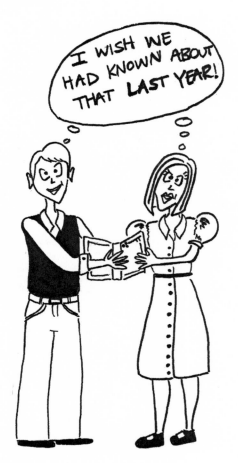

Get to Know Yourself

It is unfortunate that many people do not really know themselves very well. They have never studied what type of person they are, what they look like to others, or compared their values and beliefs with others. There are many personality profiles, skills profiles, and psychological tests you can take to learn about yourself. Perhaps even more insightful would be to ask your spouse or family members or close friends to write up your strengths and weaknesses, and also what they like about you and what areas you could work to improve. What you hear will probably be a surprise to you.

Because the child with a disability is at a natural disadvantage in dealing with the world, he will tend to use whatever he can to get attention or to get what he wants. The child will use the same ploys as other children and sometimes some unique ones. This can be anything from pouting to whining to faking illness or pain, etc. Many times the child with the disability is getting a lot more attention compared to the other children in the family. The other children will then act out to

> "What can help is to gain awareness of your own hot buttons."

get attention and to get what *they* want. What frequently happens is that this behavior can easily result in anger and frustration for you.

What can help is to gain awareness of your own hot buttons. For example, I have a hard time helping people with complex problems when all they think they want is a start. This happens when showing people how to use computer software. I sometimes get exasperated when I start to help a person and they make mental leaps about the next steps. Invariably they guess wrong and then get frustrated. I make a conscious effort not to get upset when this happens because I know how limited my frustration level can be in this particular situation.

When You Are Feeling Down

Being the parent of a child with a disability will likely lead to feeling down or even depressed. A negative response is natural in this situation for most people.

Unfortunately, when we are depressed, we tend to be a lot less fun to be around. We also have a lot less capacity to handle those hot button things we just discussed above.

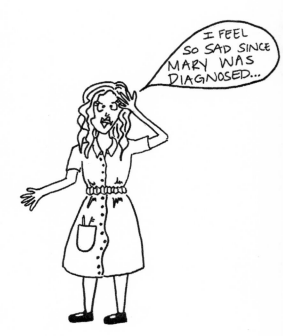

Unless you are very unusual, you will be depressed at times. The symptoms are feelings such as:

1. Loss of energy

2. Shorter temper

3. Loss of appetite

4. Difficulty in focusing

5. Lowered sex drive

6. Feeling like you are not in control of things

What causes you to be depressed? Some causes may be:

1. A lack of feeling valued because you cannot do much to help the situation (this can be really tough if you lose your job as I did a few times) or because your spouse has moved much of the focus off of your relationship to helping your child;

2. A feeling of incompetence, especially if your spouse has developed skills in helping your child that you do not have;

3. Not feeling capable of handling the situation and all you do is get angry and make things worse;

4. Not feeling worthwhile because nothing you do well seems to be what is needed;

5. In the overall situation, you do not see a light at the end of the tunnel—or if you do, it looks like a train coming and things may get worse, not better;

6. Other problems such as pressure from work that add to your feelings of being overwhelmed.

Depression will likely happen, but it should pass after a few days or a week or so. I have had short bouts of depression on a regular basis over the last three decades. For many years, I just shrugged it off as not feeling well, being down, biorhythms, allergies, etc. Only in the last ten years have I recognized that it was periods of depression. Moreover, I did not share these feelings with Gena because I did not understand them.

A great way to feel better in general is to do something to help someone else. We found that running the support group was a great way to feel better. We had many parents thank us for this effort. We have also witnessed many people learning key things that they needed to understand. Helping others is a great way to feel good about yourself, and it does not need to be directly related to your child's disability. Just doing the local walk for Cystic Fibrosis, helping once a week at the local food pantry, or doing volunteer work at a nursing home can be very rewarding. It helps others and you will definitely feel better for the experience! This is a definite win-win choice.

When you are just feeling down or feeling depressed, you are not much good to anyone—including yourself. Your lost focus means that your work will suffer, you cannot handle problems as well as you usually do, you are not much fun to be around, and you can do little to support your family. As long as this is temporary and you get back to being your old self, everyone can deal with it. More than likely, there will not be any long-term problems. Most of us can just get through these difficult times as long as they are temporary and not too painful. However, if depression tends to last more than a few days, and especially if your recovery periods are shorter than the down times, then you may need to get serious about doing something to stop it.

Serious Depression

If you are depressed a lot and the symptoms rarely go away, then you might be experiencing what is called clinical depression. This can be dangerous! Many experts believe that clinical depression is caused by a change in your body chemistry, and you cannot tough it out or just let it go on until it cures itself. *Please go see your doctor.* This is an illness, not just you feeling bad, and it will not just go away anytime soon. There are two basic treatments:

1. Antidepressant drugs

2. Psychological treatment

Many of us men do not want to go see a psychologist or psychiatrist and certainly do not want to admit that we need to take antidepressant drugs. Neither choice is very macho. However, being depressed for weeks and weeks is not very macho, either. Most men I know will resist either or both of these solutions and some men will stay depressed for years just to avoid treatment. Women can also be resistant, but our experience is that they are more likely to seek help than men.

> "Most men I know will resist either or both of these solutions and some men will stay depressed for years just to avoid treatment."

Taking the antidepressants will likely start helping you in a few weeks. Remember that clinical depression is likely caused by a *chemical imbalance* in your body and the drugs act to correct that imbalance. If you have high blood pressure, would you refuse to take medicine to reduce it? If you have high cholesterol, a high fever, or an abscessed tooth, would you refuse to take medicine or treatment? If you feel down all the time, go see your doctor. If doing the same things you have been doing is not working, then perhaps doing something different will help!

Addressing the causes of your down times and depression will generally require you to really do some soul searching with the help of family and friends or possibly professionals. When our children were young, Gena strongly encouraged us to go to a family psychologist to talk about our problems. At the time, we did not really know what was wrong with our son. He was having many learning and behavior problems at school and was in special education classes. He had the wrong diagnosis the entire time he was in school. We were all upset and frustrated a lot of the time.

I was a little resistant to seeing a psychologist. OK, I was very resistant to going to these meetings. I was embarrassed to be seeing a "shrink," even just a family shrink. However, he did help us understand why we were feeling upset, what the impact was on our daughter, and the impact on our marital relationship. With all the TV shows and general awareness about psychology, I think there are fewer stigmas now about going to get help. If you are depressed a lot, I think you are foolish not to get help. It will very likely help you to feel better, and then you can be a better parent, spouse, or friend.

Balance

There are five aspects of our lives and the balance between them is of critical importance. The five aspects are our mental lives, our social lives, our spiritual lives, our physical lives, and our emotional lives. Obviously, at any given time you can be more focused on one aspect to the exclusion of the others. If you are working out or playing a softball game, you will be focused on the physical. Taking a test, you are focused on the mental, and when attending a wedding reception, you are focused on socializing. The key is to have a good mix of all five in the life you are living.

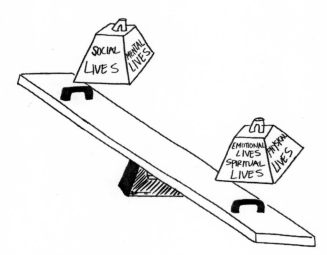

The workaholic is over focused on the mental; the athlete is frequently over focused on the physical. Many parents can be over focused on work, care giving, or their favorite sport. If things are tough in one area, we tend to avoid that area. Lots of workaholics or physical fitness nuts do too much just so they do not have to face things at home. Still others are so focused on their spiritual life that they neglect their social life and maybe their mental life and their jobs. It is OK to be highly focused, just not all the time. Ask your friends if you are in balance. They will likely know if you are skewed one way or another. Crowding out areas of your life will lead to being out of balance. Being out of balance for an extended period can easily lead to depression or other negative outcomes.

> "We need to have balance and have a part of our focus on each of these five areas of our lives."

The Bible is full of guidance on balance between the five areas. Paul calls for balance between the physical and the spiritual (1 Timothy 4:8). All the gospels talk about the social life that Jesus had with sinners and with the righteous. Jesus put his disciples in a position of great honor when He called his disciples his friends (John 15: 13-14). In Proverbs 29:11, the writer cautions us to be careful with our emotions and to be self-controlled as does Nehemiah in Nehemiah 9:17. Paul tells us to have proper control of our mental lives when he writes, "Finally, brothers whatever is true, whatever is noble, whatever is right, whatever is pure, whatever is lovely, whatever is admirable—if anything is excellent or praiseworthy—think about such things" (Philippians 4:8 NIV). We need to have balance and have a part of our focus on each of these five areas of our lives.

Educate Yourself

At the time of your child's diagnosis, illness, or accident, you will be at a disadvantage due to your lack of knowledge. Do not let the situation stay that way.

Getting yourself educated about your child's disability is perhaps the most important thing you can do to help. Becoming an expert in the disability will allow you to make better decisions and will help you to evaluate accurately the care recommendations suggested by the professionals. Who knows your child better than you and your spouse? Combining your knowledge of your child with a strong knowledge of the disability will give your child the best chance he or she will have to be successful.

> "Combining your knowledge of your child with a strong knowledge of the disability will give your child the best chance he or she will have to be successful."

For most school-age disabilities, there will be two sets of knowledge you will need to acquire. First is the medical knowledge. You need to know answers to questions like:

What is the cause of this?

What are the most common treatments and
the side effects of these treatments?

Where is the best place to get treatment?

What will it cost and who can help?

What is the likely outcome in the future?

Secondly, you will need to understand the educational diagnostic system and responses. You will need answers to questions like:

What is the educational diagnosis?

What are the school's responsibilities?

What resources does the school have and where are they?

What is the educational evaluation process?

What is an IEP and what does a good one look like?

What services will my child receive?

What is the process to have re-evaluations done and the timing of them?

How will the school and the family work together?

What can I do if I do not agree with the school's decisions?

Gena and I were at a disadvantage in our self-education as we did not have the correct diagnosis for Brent until three years *after* he graduated from high school. One of the reasons Gena started her school psychologist studies was to better understand his problems. The more she learned, the more she was able to influence the school and his treatments.

For most parents, the child's disability will have a clear label and you can research it. The Internet is a great source of information, but not all of it is accurate and it can be very confusing. For example, with autism, there are web sites that talk about many different causes and cures that sound reasonable. As of this time, there is no definitive known cause(s) for autism and many of the so-called "cures" will not work for all individuals. With a computer connected to the Internet, there is almost unlimited information available on almost any disability. I did a search for cystic fibrosis and found 1.6 million results on a search engine, 2.5 million for Attention Deficit Disorder (ADD), and 2 million for childhood diabetes.

The prudent approach is to stick to the web sites (and referrals from those sites) of the national societies for the specific disabilities of concern. These are some of the sites for major disabilities:

United Cerebral Palsy	www.ucp.org
Autism Society of America	www.autism-society.org
National Down Syndrome Society	www.ndss.org
American Association on Intellectual and Developmental Disabilities	www.aaidd.org
National Federation of the Blind	www.nfb.org
Children and Adults with ADHD	www.chadd.org
American Society for Deaf Children	www.deafchildren.org
Cystic Fibrosis Foundation	www.cff.org
Learning Disabilities	www.ncld.org
Traumatic Brain Injury	www.ninds.nih.gov/

The Federal Government also has a lot of information at the web site of the Center for Disease Control www.cdc.gov.

There is no substitute for knowledge. In dealing with caregivers, therapists, doctors, school psychologists, or teachers, it is important to know the lingo. You must know what they mean when they use words such as prognosis, behavior plan, speech or reading milestones, etc. You cannot expect to know as much as they do, but you know your child better than they ever will.

A good way to get a jump-start on your knowledge is to attend a conference focused on your child's disability. There are scores of conferences on autism, cystic fibrosis, ADD, and other major disabilities. Conferences will frequently have topics for the first time attendee as well as presentations on treatments and interventions. Parental panel discussions on the experiences of other parents are also frequently provided. Many conferences also will have a display area where books and other educational materials are available.

As previously mentioned, a great source of information is available from support groups. These groups are frequently run by professionals in the field or by a combination of parents and professionals, and will be largely attended by parents of children with the disability. Picking the brain of an experienced parent can be one of the best things you will ever do to put your situation in perspective and to get the information you are seeking (and maybe learn a few things you did not know even existed or were possible). For example, we have seen many parents shocked that the services their school system rejected for their child were available from a different school or at a different school district. Sometimes this district is adjacent to their own school district. Furthermore, just knowing that what you are going through is not unique can be very helpful.

Again, the Bible has much to say about wisdom and the value of knowledge. Ecclesiastes 7:12 (NIV) states, "Wisdom is a shelter as money is a shelter, but the advantage of knowledge is this: that wisdom preserves the life of its possessor." Proverbs 24:5 (NIV) tells us, "A wise man has great power, and a man of knowledge increases strength." Clearly, it is good to be knowledgeable, and to use that knowledge wisely. The more informed a parent is, the better decisions he will make and the better he will be able to support and help his family.

Chapter Take-a-ways:

Take care of yourself so you can take care of your family.

Have balance in your life between the mental, physical, social, spiritual, and emotional.

Learn all you can to make a positive difference.

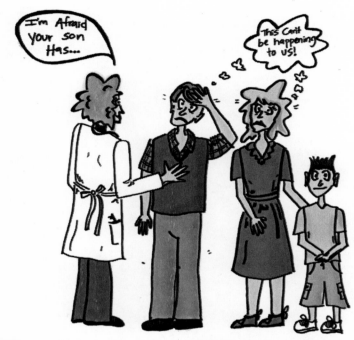

CHAPTER 10
"Mister Fix-It"

129

L et's start with a little test for fathers (this is a test I have failed many times). Can you remember the last time your wife came to you and had a problem she wanted to talk about? What were the steps that occurred? It might have gone something like this: "Honey I have this problem; can I tell you about it?" You naturally, as a good husband, say sure and start to listen. After about a minute or two you ask a clarifying question, and about two minutes later you make a small suggestion. She appears put off a bit, but she keeps on going. After about 4-5 more minutes you are pretty sure you have the problem down pat and you have two really good suggestions as to how to deal with it. So naturally, you break in and offer your ideas. These take you about 45 seconds and you stop and wait for her to thank you for your help and pick one of your solutions. The response is not exactly what you were expecting. Your wife gives you this ugly look and says, "I'll think about it," and walks off in an obviously sour mood.

What went wrong? Well, actually quite a few things. First, she has a problem, but she did not ask you to solve it; she just asked if she could talk to you about it. Regardless of the nature of the problem, it is very important to listen to what she is *actually asking for*. Second, the father in the example above did not have the patience to listen very long and get the full story. As many men do, he started to evaluate the situation almost immediately, and as she continued to talk he was only half listening. Third, his mind was already focusing on possible solutions. He was in his "mister fix-it" mode.

From a father's point of view, the scenario above makes little sense. What is not to be appreciated about a few good suggestions? Who would want to leave a problem just sitting there without some approaches for solving the problem? Why can't we discuss ways to actually solve the problem? Well, many people just want to bounce the ideas off someone. It helps them to organize their thinking and to put things in perspective. They may or may not want answers, but they do want full attention and time to get all of their thoughts presented. Coming up with answers or suggestions

> "They may or may not want answers, but they do want full attention and time to get all of their thoughts presented."

is not what they want at this time. When they have fully talked themselves out, then your ideas and suggestions may be very much appreciated—or maybe not.

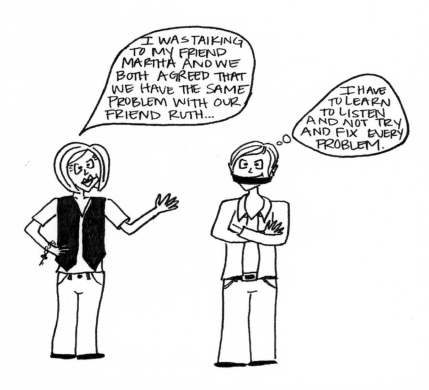

Parents of Children with Disabilities

While I have used the husband and wife scenario above, clearly this applies to many situations such as meetings at work, meetings with school personnel, social conversations, and especially in interactions with your children. This type of situation also can be reversed with the husband wanting to talk and the spouse half listening and making suggestions. As your children approach their teens, they will be less and less interested in your solutions to their problems and more and more interested in verifying that *you care enough to just listen.* If they ask for your ideas, feel free to give them, but hold off if you can when they just want to talk.

Frustrated Mister Fix-It

You have probably tried many things to help your child and your family deal with the challenges of your child's disability. It is not unusual for parents to try different doctors, different therapies and therapists, different medications, different schools, etc. These are all admirable efforts to at least partially fix the situation. However, if after a lot of time, money, and effort the child still cannot walk, still cannot talk, or still is severely disabled, then frustration will set in. You cannot seem to fix it no matter what you try. You do not want to admit defeat, but the evidence is staring you right in the face every day.

Part of the problem may be that you have not accepted the disability. You may not be willing to accept the child as he or she is and will do everything in your power to change him or her. Check your motives here. Are you doing all this for the child or for yourself? Is it really so tragic for the child or for you that he or she will be dealing with the disability all of his or her life?

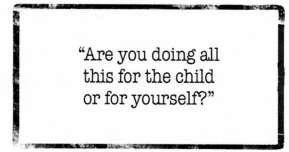

"Are you doing all this for the child or for yourself?"

Another problem for the "mister fix-it" is when someone else is able to fix something that you have not been successful at fixing. A classic example is when the spouse comes up with a solution that you did not think of—and it works. Even more humbling is when one of your other children solves a problem you've been working on for a long time. A great example of this is the story of a father trying to train his child with Down syndrome to ride a bike. Try as he could, the child was just not willing to go fast enough to balance the bike. Big sister on her own took her brother out one day, and the brother conquered his fear and was able to ride the bike. Similar situations can arise in toilet training, teaching a child math or reading, etc. The brother or sister or one of the parents may have a unique relationship and ability to communicate that gives him or her a real advantage in helping. They may also be able to motivate in an entirely different way. It can be humbling, but trying to always be "mister fix-it" can be an unsuccessful approach.

Children with neurological disorders, such as our son with Asperger Syndrome, are not able to take suggestions well at times. Our son was 29 years old when he had some lower back and leg pain on and off for a few weeks. A muscle relaxant had not solved the problem and I suggested that he call the doctor and get an appointment that day, instead of waiting until next week for his scheduled follow-up appointment. It seemed like a no brainer to me, but he said he "would think about it." That was a Friday and I could not understand why he would stay in pain over the weekend. As of 1:40 in the afternoon, he was still thinking about it. I could have tried to force him to go. I could have called the doctor for him, but if he didn't want to go, was I really fixing the problem? He may go but be very resentful of me forcing him to do something he did not want to do. Late in the day, he finally did go and got some help.

Another aspect of this same problem is that the normal issues that arise in dealing with children are magnified with a disability. Medication can pose problems if there are a number of different medications involved. Interactions between the medications can become a serious concern. A new medication or treatment has to be viewed in the context of the overall treatments being used.

Costs are usually pretty significant, and family budgets and family time can be severely impacted. Sometimes when we try to fix one problem it just creates a new problem. Many times it is like squeezing a balloon between your fingers. If you squeeze one part it just pops out somewhere else!

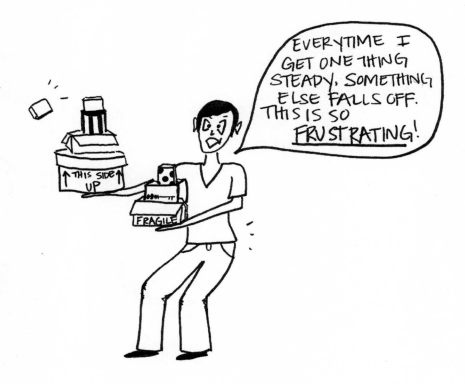

For example, assume that there is a strain on the family budget because of medications or therapy or the spouse cannot work because of the needs of the child. One solution is for you to take a second part-time job or to work more overtime. Maybe you work retail one weekend day and two weekday nights. That helps solve the money problem, but now you are away from the home a lot more and your spouse gets less relief. The increased stress just makes things that much less pleasant and everyone in the family suffers.

Some Suggestions

Many fathers and mothers tend to have strong egos when it comes to solving problems. Many of us are "results oriented" people. We will tackle a problem logically in an organized fashion and put together a plan. It may even have milestones and target results for steps along the way. Fathers especially will frequently put a lot of energy and focus into solving a problem. We will take "ownership" of the problem and "ownership" of the solution. Generally, this is well and good. A strong, logical, forceful approach to problem solving is frequently the only way to solve a difficult and/or complex problem. We can even use our anger and frustration to help us focus our efforts and add energy to the effort.

One problem that I have seen is when other family members make suggestions or recommendations, or outright question the parent's approach to solving the problem. If the problem is a persistent one and the father's solution is not working very well, then suggestions sound a lot like criticism and the parent can easily feel resentful and incompetent. This feels like an attack on the whole approach to dealing with problems.

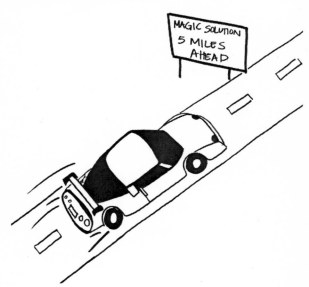

Treating a disability is usually the role of doctors and specialists. When a parent has tried his or her best and been unsuccessful, perhaps it is worth reviewing their role. Most parents are not doctors or specialists. They may know their child better than anyone, but they are generally not educated and trained enough to properly treat the disability. Many times parents will focus on a single approach when a multi-step approach will work better. Sometimes, it seems they will do almost anything to try to fix the situation. Again, I urge you to review your motives and proceed with caution. Some of the solutions can be very expensive and even dangerous to the child.

There is also a tendency for other family members and your well-intentioned friends to push you to consider their "pet ideas" on how to solve the problem. This can be very distracting. In addition, if you do not follow their advice, your friends and family members can feel slighted and unappreciated. Children without obvious physical disabilities, such as Asperger Syndrome or mild intellectual disability, will frequently be labeled by the uninformed as just lazy or as not trying hard enough. You may even get requests from people (usually relatives) to take your child for a week with an offer of "We will straighten them out!" There is the clear judgment that you are an incompetent parent and some solid discipline will make all the difference. While no one should even consider such an offer, it places you in a situation where you have to be strong to say, "No thank you." Rarely is there a simple or obvious solution. Strength and patience are needed here to protect yourself and your family.

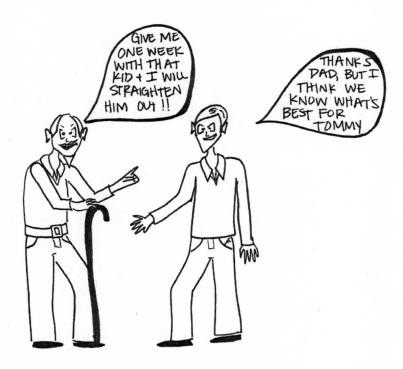

Giving Up

A common result of the on-going frustration of a permanent disability is that the parent will have a tendency to give up. All the "solutions" and the "fixes" have not worked. All the "help" from family and friends has just made things seem worse. The parent may just give up trying. What's the point of beating yourself against the wall on this? Fathers especially may then become angry because of the continued frustration, or they may just withdraw and push themselves as far away from the situation as they can get. Clearly, this is not what is best for the family. There is nothing much worse than an angry parent or a totally withdrawn parent. Neither is doing anything positive to help the situation. If you find yourself in this situation, please read the chapter Helping Yourself.

Working to fix things is not bad. There is nothing wrong with trying to do well, to make things better for others and for yourself. The ancient words of the 112th Psalm verses 4-9 (NLT) certainly support this:

Light shines in the darkness for the godly.

They are generous, compassionate, and righteous.

Good comes to those who lend money generously
and conduct their business fairly.

Such people will not be overcome by evil.

Those who are righteous will be long remembered.

They do not fear bad news; they confidently
trust the LORD to care for them.

They are confident and fearless and can face their foes triumphantly.

They share freely and give generously to those in need.
Their good deeds will be remembered forever.

They will have influence and honor.

Clearly the good works of the righteous will be rewarded and will lead to positive outcomes for you and for your family. Giving your time and energy generously to those in need is most honorable and rewarding. A word of caution however, from Proverbs 19:2 (NLT): "Zeal without knowledge is not good; a person who moves too quickly may go the wrong way." Trying to fix things and trying to do good is not enough. You must have the knowledge and skills to do it *right*. A realistic view of what we know and what we can realistically accomplish is true wisdom. Patience is essential if you are not sure you are on the correct path to solving a problem.

We also read that when bad things happen, help will be on the way. It may not always be what we think we want or need, but light will come bursting in. Light is a reference to wisdom. The "light" the good receive may not be a solution or a godly fix, but may instead be better understanding or insight. It might also be that what you learn can be of great help to your family, to yourself, and to others facing a similar situation. Clearly, bad things happen to all people, those good and bad. True wisdom also may be accepting things as they are and doing the best we can do. A permanent disability is not likely to be miraculously cured. The difficul-

> "A realistic view of what we know and what we can realistically accomplish is true wisdom."

ties may continue, and there may be no way to fix them. Nevertheless, good can come out of the situation, if you are wise in what you do to help. This book is an example of good that can come from a difficult situation.

Chapter Take-a-ways:

Learn to listen and get the whole story before suggesting solutions.

Some problems are not fixable and the lesson may involve acceptance.

Be patient in trying new solutions,
but keep working to help others and your children.

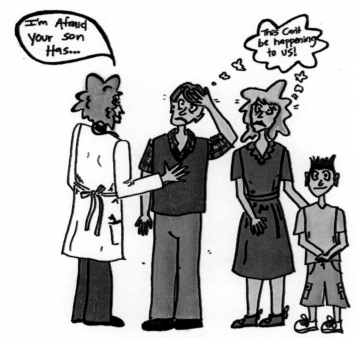

CHAPTER 11

Carl's Story

141

T he year 1986 proved to be very memorable for two reasons. At the age of 27 (long after my mother had given up hope), I finally found someone to share my life with and was married. At the same time, I accepted God's call to ministry. Little did I know at the time how closely the two would be connected.

The following year, Vicki and I left Wichita for Florida where we became active in a good church and started our life together. A year and a half later our first child, David, was born. It was a difficult labor but at 9 pounds and 6 ounces and with all fingers and toes present, life was good. Just over a year after that, Stephen joined us following an uneventful pregnancy and incredibly easy labor. It appeared that all was still well.

However, as Stephen progressed, it became clear that he was different. All the critical milestones occurred on schedule; sitting, crawling, standing, walking, potty training, etc. Yet something was still very different. From a very early age, Stephen would wake up at night and play by himself for hours without making any noise. This habit continues even now at sixteen. Stephen was always preoccupied with order and neatness. I love cooking and will often be in the kitchen with all the cupboards and drawers open at once. As soon as Stephen started walking he would follow me around and close everything behind me. A development screening at 14 months noted his fixation with stacking blocks. Stephen would stack blocks until they fell, erupt in rage, and then start over. This behavior would continue for hours.

Possibly the most unusual of Stephen's behaviors was his physical contact with other people. With few exceptions, Stephen has always been and continues to be upset by other people touching him. Vicki and I, his grandmothers, and a few teachers are the only people he has ever opened up to. Even then he has to feel like he is in control of the situation. At age two, Stephen developed a ritual of waiting till we were seated, lifting our shirt, turning around and facing the other way, then backing up to us, taking our hands and wrapping our arms around him.

Many thought Stephen had a hearing loss because he would often act as though he didn't hear people speaking to him. At other times I could whisper his name from across the room and have him respond. Language development was also seriously delayed. At age three he had a vocabulary of only about 50 words. It was at this point we decided to have him evaluated for admission into an early childhood education program. Hearing and vision tests showed no problems. A medical exam showed no physical problems. Developmental tests showed some abnormalities but in the early 90s psychologists were not looking for autism except in the most severe cases. He clearly had language delays so the evaluating psychologist finally summarized Stephen with the statement, "He has some problems with language but give him a couple of years of special education and he will be fine."

It was about this time that we noticed a new problem appearing. During his first three years of life, Stephen had been fairly isolated, only having regular contact with close family. Vicki stayed home with the boys. Our church nursery was very small. Most social situations were centered around family. But now school, church, and other social activities forced Stephen into close contact with many more people. He would try to isolate himself and was subject to very strong outbursts. Trying to control his actions in public settings often turned into a battle. During his two years of early childhood education, most days degenerated into Stephen grabbing a few toys, diving under a corner table, and fighting off anyone who tried to make him move. It would be three more years before we would learn what caused these reactions and how we could best manage them.

One particularly bad day during this period was destined to change my life. A year after Stephen was born, I enrolled in seminary to complete my education. Receiving my Masters in religious education in 1993, I accepted a position as educational minister in a small church. One Sunday, Stephen was having a very difficult day. There was a potluck dinner in the evening and I stayed at the table with Vicki to help control him. The next day I was called and told that, "...my job was to do church business. If Vicki could not control Stephen, they were both welcome to stay home." It was then that I realized Stephen is my son and my ministry. His well-being will always come first with me. Any church that fails to welcome my child doesn't want me, either. For several years that meant that the two of us stayed home most Sunday mornings. Luckily, we have now found a church where Stephen is welcome "as is."

> "Any church that fails to welcome my child doesn't want me, either."

This has continued to be a touchy subject with me over the years. The reality is very few churches are really willing to accept people with developmental or physical disabilities. When the Americans with Disabilities Act (ADA) was passed in 1990, many churches were vocal in their opposition to being "forced" to comply with its provisions. I'm sorry but I really believe churches should be leading the fight for accessibility. Repeatedly in the gospels, we read of men and women coming to Jesus for healing whose paths were blocked by well-meaning disciples. Jesus never failed to admonish any who would attempt to shut out these individuals. He accepted everybody "as is." How would He feel about churches that block the path of those who are "different"?

Stephen's entry into the school environment brought a new set of challenges. At the forefront were IEP meetings. Today, many minor changes can be made without a formal IEP meeting but when Stephen started school nothing could change without a meeting. Written notices had to be sent to all participants. Each meeting required us to be presented with yet another printed copy of our rights and responsibilities. And each meeting required an entirely new IEP to be written. Once a year was bad enough but one year we were having a meeting every month. I am glad that today we can interact less formally and get results faster.

Elementary School

After two years of early childhood education, Stephen entered kindergarten. His teacher, Mrs. M, was an experienced classroom teacher who was starting her first year of special education. Our district keeps students in elementary special education with the same teacher each year so she and Stephen were to be together for most of the next six years. I won't hesitate in saying that this arrangement is what set the stage for much of Stephen's success in school. Mrs. M was the first teacher who explored beyond Stephen's labels (language delay, behavior disorder) and searched for a cause. The following year, she enrolled in a graduate program in autism in order to learn more about working with students with this disorder. Stephen quickly bonded with Mrs. M and they remained close for his entire time in elementary school.

That doesn't mean that there weren't problems. Stephen was still subject to violent outbursts and would try to run away from school when he was unhappy with a decision. I was called to come pick him up many times. He remained largely non-verbal and was very difficult to understand when he did speak. As three years had passed since his initial evaluation, a re-evaluation was scheduled. It was apparent that the initial evaluation was off-target. Two years of language assistance hadn't solved his problems. After a couple weeks of testing, we started meeting with the team members. It was while going over the results of his assessments that the school psychologist asked us if we had considered whether Stephen might be autistic. My first response was "no way." Stephen didn't match the pictures I had seen of children with autism. Besides, if that was the case, why hadn't anyone mentioned it before? I have discovered in the years since that many families spend years before getting a correct diagnosis. I know one woman whose 13-year-old son was just diagnosed after being labeled ADD, behavior disorder, and several other misdiagnoses. Luckily for us, the school psychologist (Gena Barnhill, the co-author) was going through the same thing with her son. She helped us to understand that autism has many forms and directed us to the resources we needed to get a conclusive diagnosis.

In the summer of 1997, Stephen started a complete medical evaluation. Luckily I had a job that allowed very flexible work schedules. After our initial appointment with a psychiatrist, tests were ordered to rule out other possibilities. An EEG indicated some possible abnormalities which led to a follow-up MRI and referral to a neurologist. In the meantime, all kinds of IQ, behavioral, and developmental tests were being conducted. The final conclusion was that Stephen had several congenital brain abnormalities that might be causing his autism. That's the fun thing about autism — we don't know what causes it, we don't know who will get it, and we don't know how to get rid of it. The final diagnosis was PDD-NOS which is a catch-all for those cases where the experts aren't quite sure that it is autism. It took another eight years before a re-evaluation clearly indicated autism.

Both the psychiatrist and neurologist recommended pharmaceutical treatment for Stephen's symptoms. He was prescribed a combination of Zoloft and Depakote. The Depakote sent him through the roof so he was moved to Tegretol instead. The effects were pretty immediate. Stephen's rage episodes nearly disappeared. He appeared much more able to handle school and public situations. Over the next several years, Stephen's teachers were able to work with him on handling social situations and he has improved greatly. We are now trying to see if he can function without the drugs.

Middle School

The stability of elementary school unfortunately did not carry over into middle school. As in elementary, middle school students are kept together as a group.

However, in three years, Stephen had three different teachers due to staff turnover. Only one of the three is still involved in special education. This made carrying out IEP goals and long-term plans very difficult. Each year we spent valuable time explaining things to new staff. Sadly, this is all too common in special education. Until we begin to adequately fund and support special education, it is unlikely to change. Stephen did well academically during these three years. He is an avid reader with a near-photographic memory. Stephen often surprises people with his ability to quickly grasp new material. Social interaction was a little harder, though. While he quickly learned to maneuver the hallways, Stephen did not know how to appropriately approach and interact with others. He would step on a teacher's toes to get her attention or stand immediately behind someone and expect them to acknowledge him.

High School

Stephen's entry into high school has gone remarkably well. The school holds classes on alternating days. Early on, this lead to some confusion and he would show up in the wrong room. I pick one class he really likes from each day's schedule and just remind him each morning which of those classes he will have that day. Knowing that helps him keep track of the rest of his schedule. Stephen is primarily involved in structured classes that accommodate his needs for extra time, etc. Next year he will begin spending some time each day in developing the ability to move into the workforce upon graduation.

Changes in My Life

This year has also been one of change for me. As well as Stephen does in school, he functions on a very low level when it comes to self-care. In many ways it is like having a five- or six-year-old. Stephen was 15 before he could tie his shoes. He still needs reminders and assistance with grooming, bathing, and medicine. Unless reminded regularly, Stephen will forget his address, phone number, and age. He has no sense of danger and regularly opens the door to any knock. In re-

Parents of Children with Disabilities

> "As a result, I moved to a part-time job with the school district last year so I could be home whenever Stephen is not in school."

ality, Stephen cannot be left alone for any length of time. This will probably always be the case. Recently, I was going over rules for staying home alone with Stephen. We discussed ignoring the door if someone knocked and ignoring the phone if it rang. I then asked him what he would do if the house was on fire. His answer was, "Ignore it."

Our oldest son has been the babysitter for many years. But he now has a job, girlfriend, and all the other trappings of a life. As a result, I moved to a part-time job with the school district last year so I could be home whenever Stephen is not in school. It has also given me time to deal with applying for SSI, fighting state agencies, scheduling evaluations, and becoming Stephen's life-skills teacher. It has also given me more time to help my wife. She has always had trouble handling spoken conversation and being in crowds. As a child she was labeled a problem learner. Later the diagnoses were auditory processing disorder and ADD. However, none of the standard treatments helped. This past year I have been studying adolescent and adult autism in order to better understand Stephen's progress. It became clear that as Stephen aged, they were sharing many traits. Several months ago, she was diagnosed as having a very high functioning form of autism. Now that she has an accurate diagnosis we are able to learn together how to better help her function.

A lot of my identity went into being the bread-winner and it hasn't been easy dropping to 1/3 of my former salary. It has taken a lot of cutting and downward mobility to make it work so far. I don't

> "A lot of my identity went into being the bread-winner and it hasn't been easy dropping to 1/3 of my former salary."

know how long this arrangement will last but for now it is giving Stephen what he needs.

Twelve years of school down—three more to go. Sometimes it has been great. At other times it has been incredibly frustrating. Even with good teachers and support staff, I have never been able to sit back and stop fighting for even a moment. As I mentioned earlier, Stephen has a near-photographic memory. He memorizes building layouts and schedules. This has often led his teachers to believe that he is functioning "normally." By fourth grade, Stephen had been in the same classroom for five years and had the routine memorized. The IEP meeting was held just before the end of school. His teacher came to the conclusion that Stephen was showing little sign of autism and had no need for Extended School Year (ESY) services. Nothing would change her mind. I finally had to demand that Stephen be removed from all special education services and be transferred to the school he would have normally attended. That forced the district to conduct a re-assessment. The results clearly showed that Stephen was not functioning as well as indicated by classroom behavior. All services, including ESY, were reinstated. Stephen has severe coordination problems. At the last IEP of middle school, we specified no shop classes and no regular PE classes in high school. When Stephen and I went to enroll for high school, he had been scheduled for both woodworking and regular PE in his first semester. Luckily, this time a quick meeting set everything straight.

In twelve years I have learned the system—what buttons to push, where to complain, and where to compliment. I don't expect much trouble in the next three years. But the future does worry me. I don't think school districts and staff are evil. Most are just overworked and under-supported. However, the rules are changing. More of the burden of proof is being placed on the family today. Traditionally, if a district denied services, it had the burden of proof to show why. Now if a family wants to fight a denial they can be forced to prove that the initial decisions were in error. Very few families have the time or resources to secure the evaluations and expert opinions that would be needed. That means more and more of our children will be languishing without the services they need to make progress.

Another thing that worries me is adulthood. In less than two years, my relationship with Stephen will change. I will still be his father but my role will be changed. The law says he will make his own decisions then unless I have him publicly declared incompetent to make decisions. I don't know how others handle it but the thought of going to a stranger and asking them to formally declare my son to be helpless bothers me. I have fought to make others see what Stephen has inside. Now I have to try and hide those qualities. Many families are able to use a power-of-attorney to allow decision making to be shared. With Stephen, I will need to file for guardianship and make all his decisions. I also have to start looking at how Stephen will continue to function when I am not around. In order to avoid jeopardizing any benefits he might be receiving, special trusts must be set up and funded. An alternate guardian must be appointed and prepared. With most children this isn't too involved. But with Stephen, I need to document his complete medical history, every condition and medicine, his habits and quirks, likes and dislikes. In essence, I have to write a handbook to train his next caregiver should they be needed.

The greatest fear for most men is being forced to admit they don't have everything under control. For the fathers of children with disabilities, it is a normal state of affairs. Most days I feel overwhelmed. I can't make Stephen better; most of the time I can't even get him the services or appointments he needs. I know that I too frequently rely on my oldest son to take care of himself. I don't know if I am providing enough support to my wife but I know we don't get enough time together. Since qualified babysitters don't exist here, our lives and work schedules

> "The greatest fear for most men is being forced to admit they don't have everything under control. For the fathers of children with disabilities, it is a normal state of affairs."

revolve around taking care of Stephen. That arrangement will not change for years, if ever. Statistically 75-80% of families having children with disabilities end up divorcing. So far we have beat the odds but we don't underestimate how stressful it will be. I don't know how to cut back on work and at the same time fund his future care. Don't ask about our retirement because I haven't even started working on it. Sometimes nothing works and frustration gets the best of me. Luckily I have found a church community that holds me up both spiritually and emotionally.

Things I Have Learned

Press' plans for this chapter were to deal with success stories. I am not sure as I write this paragraph if my story fits. Most days I am glad to simply survive. But there are some lessons that have become clear over the years. The first is that no job can serve as my identity. I have walked away from two career positions because they demanded more time than I could share. My calling is as parent and caregiver. Jobs are tools that help me perform my calling but they are never the calling. The second lesson is that I cannot let my family become my entire identity either. Ignoring my own needs only lessens my ability to meet their needs. I have to take care of myself physically, mentally, and spiritually. I frequently have to step back and remind myself of this. I can only urge you to take time and find your own interests.

Make sure you create and nurture close friendships. We were not created to be loners. Some of the greatest stories in the Bible center on the power of friendship. I recently read a book on prayer as a dialogue between friends. It helps to be reminded I have a friend who is always close by. Don't be

> "The first lesson is that no job can serve as my identity. I have walked away from two career positions because they demanded more time than I could share."

afraid to go beyond friendship and seek professional help. There will be times when the feeling of being overwhelmed will become overwhelming itself. This isn't how we planned our lives and there is nothing we can do to change it. That's hard to accept and I need to vent about it sometimes. Counselors are really just trained listeners. They have to sit and listen to what my friends and family may not want to hear. Support groups are composed of people who are feeling the same things you feel. It is not weakness to need that sometimes.

Finally, be a fighter. All parents are called to fight for their children but the parent of a child with a disability will be forced to fight every day. Schools, doctors, government agencies, and especially those who would shut your child out are your opponents. Learn everything you can about your child's disability. Use every resource that is available; support groups, medical literature, Internet resources, the library, classes, and most importantly those who are already doing what you want to do. Be steadfast in your commitment, seek to educate the ignorant, and don't forget to support your fellow warriors—spouse, family, teachers, case managers, and support group members.

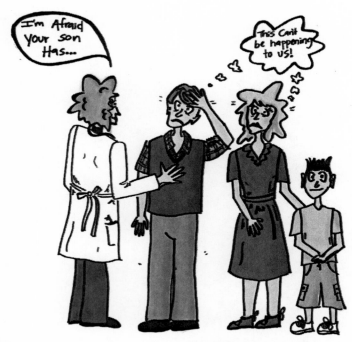

CHAPTER 12

Love, Circumstances, & Growth

155

T his was perhaps the most difficult chapter to write. To start, answer this question:

Why do we need to understand the

word love and the various forms of love?

The short answer is that we all love, and want to be loved, but most of us do not really know what love means and why the word has so many different uses and meanings. To many of us, love is a feeling or an emotion. I would argue that this is false. I believe that love is more of a decision and a commitment than an emotion. We can say we love our spouse or we love our parents. We can say we love to eat and we love God. We can say we love our sister and we love to work out at the gym. We can say we love our children. Each of these is a really different use of the word love. An Internet search on the topic "types of love" yielded 7.9 million results. So what does the word love really mean?

"I believe that love is more of a decision and a commitment than an emotion."

The Eight Types of Love

While I cannot claim to be an expert on love, I have organized the concept of love into eight different categories, and put them in alphabetical order so it is easier to remember:

A. **Agape Love**—The word agape is a word from ancient Greek and stands for love as a decision or volitional love. This is the type of love where we decide to love someone or something—not because it is merited but because we choose to love. A good example of this is when we choose to love someone who has seriously wronged us.

B. **Brotherly Love**—Most of us have a clear understanding of brotherly love or love for a friend or brother. We can "love" our brother or our friend. This type of love is usually based on a long-term relationship and is based on mutual trust and familiarity. A good understanding of each other and the ability to share honestly over time develops from a friendship into brotherly love. A good example of this type of love is that found between nuns and monks or fraternity brothers.

C. **Commitment Love**—This type of love is one many of us are familiar with—the love of family. This is based on the group relationship we have developed. The difference between brotherly love and commitment love can be explained as the difference between supporting your sister even though you do not have a close relationship. You will do whatever she needs out of commitment, not out of a close relationship. You would protect her, help her financially, help her move, and intercede in any confrontations she was facing. You would do this because you are her brother and she is part of your family.

D. **Demanding Love**—This is a very different type of love in which a person demands love from another. Some people can become very possessive of another and say they "love" in the sense that they deserve to be loved by another. This type of love is jealous, possessive, and frequently creates a dependent relationship. People can take this type of love and use it as an excuse to abuse the other person if they feel in any way that the person is not devoted to them. Many people will confuse a marriage commitment with this type of love. The spouse may assume that once he or she is married, their mate is fully committed regardless of how the relationship develops or falls apart.

E. **Erotic Love**—This is the form of love that the movies and television frequently portray. The term evolves from the Greek word Eros and is characterized by high intensity, physical and sexual connotations, and a high level of commitment on the part of both parties. This type of love is the romantic love we see in entertainment. It is the most dramatic form of love, but by its very nature is likely to last a limited time. It is just too intense and requires too much effort to keep it going. Erotic love can be a wonderful way to start a marriage, but must evolve into a different form of love to be sustainable. Unfortunately the media tend to neglect this evolution of erotic love and, to increase the entertainment value, frequently turn the relationship into something horrible such as abuse and/or murder.

F. **Friendship Love**—This is the love we develop for a friend. This usually will take many years to develop but will not be as deep or long lasting as brotherly love. Usually it is a relationship with the same sex and will not have romantic or erotic characteristics. Friendship love can develop into brotherly love if given enough time and mutual interest.

G. **Godly Love**—This is the love that God has for us. In the Bible, God's love is shown in many ways such as love for the nation of Israel, love and commitment for the Jewish race, and love for individuals such as David and Solomon. God's love is not based on what people do. God's love is unconditional, unselfish, and is given to all regardless of how we act. God's love is the perfect love we all should strive for.

H. **Happy Love**—This is the type of temporary "love" we have for another person. It is no strings attached love that lives for the moment. Children can have puppy love and young adults can have a summer love. Older adults can have a fling. It is just for fun love that is effortless and will die once any real effort or commitment is required. Rarely is this type of love more than a brief emotional high followed by a much longer emotional low.

These are the many different types of love. Unfortunately, the English language has only one word for love and this one word is used to represent all of the types of love. No wonder we are confused by the word. As shown above, real love is rarely what we see on television or at the movies. It is based on a relationship and a decision that we make. Emotions come and go, and emotions go up and down. True love is long lasting and steady, and cannot therefore be based only on emotions. It requires commitment—a commitment that goes beyond our emotions and feelings.

Parents and Love

Parents can experience love in many different ways as described above. For some parents, loving the child with a disability can be difficult. The child may have terrible behavior, be angry, be withdrawn, or even unresponsive. It can be really hard to love some children.

Likewise, being a person with a disability is not fun. People with disabilities generally cannot do many things that others can. Life is much more difficult and stressful. Given a choice, very few people with a disability would be unwilling to give up their disability. The disability forces many to be dependent on others. Children are already very dependent on their parents, but a child with a disability is even more dependent and therefore has a greater need of time and support and love. As the children and the parents age, the relationship has to change.

An adult with a disability can be similar to a teenager. The teen years are really tough for the children and for the parents. The dependency relationship is changing, but the child is not ready to be on his or her own. When a disability is involved, the child will have a more difficult time breaking away from the home or from dependence on others. In our situation, our son is 33, but has the emotional maturity of a mid-teen. He was frustrated by not being on his own, but knew he needed a lot of support. As this drags on, the child and the parent can get really tired and worn out. This is when agape love or commitment love becomes a critical approach. The parent has to decide to love or stay committed to love even as the situation is difficult with no end in sight. This is easier said than done!

> "Children are already very dependent on their parents, but a child with a disability is even more dependent and therefore has a greater need of time and support and love."

Your child deserves to be loved for who he is. The child does not have to be apologetic for being disabled, as it is almost never his fault. Everyone wants to be loved and loved for who they are. Not being loved because he is not the son we want him to be is cruel and unfair. So many of us focus on what could have been, and what the child would be like without the disability. In most cases, the disability is now part of who the child is. The child deserves to be loved *just as he or she is.* This love should be without conditions or restrictions. An emotional

> "The child deserves to be loved just as he or she is. This love should be without conditions or restrictions."

type of love cannot likely survive this. It has to be a decision to love and a commitment to love.

One of our more difficult experiences was when we were in a Bible study group that decided everyone would share great or interesting things about their children. This was generally a positive experience for most of the parents. When our turn came, we had a hard time as our great and interesting things were so different than others. To be honest, it was embarrassing and we were hurt by the experience. It just hammered home the significance of the disability and forced us to realize that our expectations were so much lower than those of the rest of the group. This negative thought pattern is not helpful in developing a loving relationship.

The ideal love is God's love. Love without conditions is something to strive for but must be tempered with the reality that we are limited in our ability to love. For most parents, the type of love we have for our children is either agape love or commitment love, or possibly some mixture of the two. No matter how you look at it though, the child deserves to be loved. You brought the child into your world. He or she needs to be loved just as the child is, not as we wanted him or her to be.

It's Not Fair!

Unfortunately, there are some parents that really do not love their child. They feel that the disability is unfair (to them) and therefore they cannot commit to the relationship. This is not what they bargained for when they decided to have children. Many parents, especially fathers we have met, feel that they have been cheated. They thought they were getting a child they could nurture and help grow into someone they could be proud of and carry on the family name. Instead, they find themselves working very hard just to take care of basic needs. Love takes effort, time, energy, and focus. They also may think that there is little point in putting great effort into achieving limited goals. This makes it difficult to move themselves to agape love. The decision to love is just too hard and the rewards are just too little.

Let's assume that this really is an unfair situation. Who is it unfair to? To the child, for sure. To the parents, for sure. To the other children, for sure. To the grandparents and the extended family, for sure. To the school system and all others who have to do extra things to help out, for sure. *It is not fair to anyone.* If you do not think you can love your child with a disability, then you need to do some soul searching. Love does not mean you have to be emotionally attached to the child. What it does mean is that you need to have agape or commitment love for your child. It is a very important decision you need to make that is fair to you and to your family.

No Pain No Gain

Let's now assume for a moment that your child is not disabled. He or she can do many of the things you hoped for when the child first arrived. Life is sweeter and easier and you can be proud of his or her accomplishments. So it is easy to love. Are you a better person because you have not had the hardship of raising a child with disabilities? I would contend that the old adage of "no pain no gain" is very relevant here. I am a much stronger and better person because of what I have had to do in raising our son. The ancient wisdom of Solomon is written so well in Proverbs 14:23a (NIV): "All hard work brings a profit." Raising a child with disabilities forces us to grow and to work harder. This builds our character and makes us stronger just as working out at the gym builds our physical strength.

There is a very mature and wonderful way to approach your situation. Some parents grow to the point that they love the child for what the child's disability has pushed them to become. Some parents have learned to accept their child's disability as a gift. I cannot honestly say I am there yet, but I am moving in that direction. Both of our lives are very different and in many ways better because of our son. We are stronger in many ways. Gena's career was changed by our son's disability and my life's work is changed to helping others instead of corporate success. This never would have happened if Brent had not been disabled.

One interesting thought is that this challenge you have been given was given for a purpose. God could have given the child with special needs to someone

> "Maybe, just maybe, you have been chosen for a special child to be a blessing to the child and to become the person God created you to be."

else. Why you? It could be because God knows you can handle it. He trusts you with His child who needs the extra care and time and energy. One of my favorite phrases is, "If it was easy, anyone could do it." Maybe, just maybe, you have been chosen for a special child to be a blessing to the child and to become the person God created you to be. You have no idea who you might become if you persevere and grow from your experiences.

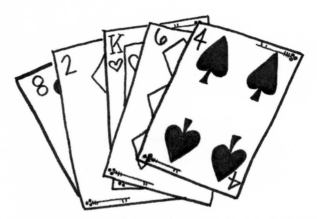

USE THE CARDS THAT HAVE BEEN DEALT TO YOU.

What's in the Cards?

Another way to look at this is to accept that you need to play with the hand that has been dealt to you. You may wish that you are getting full houses or flushes, but the reality is very different. What fun would it be to play a game you always won? Without challenges, there is no growth. Why do so many wealthy, privileged, and unchallenged people end up with meaningless lives? Without failure, there is little appreciation for success. If everything was easy, we would all be weak and never develop ourselves into the persons we can be. Be careful asking for a new set of cards. Things just might be worse, not better.

Who Do You Admire?

If you look at people you admire, I am willing to bet that each one of them went through rough times that helped them develop the very skills that you admire in them. All great football, tennis, golf, baseball, etc., players had to develop their skills by being challenged. All great leaders suffered failures and disappointments in their lives. President Lincoln is famous for all the electoral defeats and personal challenges that led to his election as president. These are growth opportunities, a way we are forced to develop our capacity and perseverance. Of course we are not claiming it is fun to be challenged and forced to change and grow. Our parents, teachers, and others taught us and disciplined us as a way to help us change our behavior.

> "Developing your ability to give true, committed love is a wonderful gift for you, for your spouse, and for your children."

Our current situation is just another form of discipline that we need to deal with to strengthen ourselves to become the best parents we can be. Avoiding this is no way to become the person that you want to be and the person that others are counting on you becoming. Developing your ability to give true, committed love is a wonderful gift for you, for your spouse, and for your children.

By the way, we know many parents who are extremely disappointed by their children that do not have disabilities. Just because a child is not disabled does not mean all will be wonderful. Many criminals, drug addicts, and people who have made a mess of their lives are not disabled. Talk about huge embarrassment and dashed expectations for these parents! If you have always wished your child were not disabled, be careful what you wish for. Things could be a lot worse, and they could be a lot harder to love than they are now.

Chapter Take-a-ways:

Be committed.

Love others the best you can.

Learn and grow from your experiences.

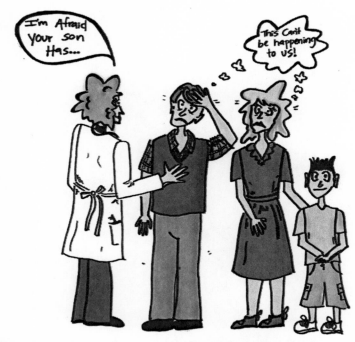

CHAPTER 13
Tyler & Becky's Story

167

"When Our World Shatters"
Tyler

I t happened suddenly without any signs or warnings. My 11-year-old son was in the hospital recovering from a severe brain hemorrhage and stroke. Aside from actually losing a child, this is undoubtedly a parent's worst nightmare. I was in a state of shock for many months. The world as I knew it no longer existed; I was desperately looking for solid ground on which to stand.

I wanted to believe that God was in the midst of the darkness that surrounded me. Four days after it happened, I wrote in my journal: "Dear Lord, I do not see; I cannot see with my eyes any light, anything to hope for. I pray, give me eyes of faith to pierce the shadow and see the evidence of things unseen."[1] That is what faith is, right? "Now faith is the substance of things hoped for, the evidence of things not seen" (Heb 11:1). And I know, at least in my mind, that God promises to "never leave us, or forsake us" (Heb 13:5). But none of these truths that I took for granted seemed to register. Rather, they seemed like empty words, as vacuous as the way I felt.

Until that night, I didn't realize how quickly one's world can be turned upside down. It wasn't like our family was a stranger to trials and hardships. I have been sick most of my adult life with a chronic lung condition; my father-in-law and brother-in-law died unexpectedly within a period of two years; we have moved nine times in nineteen years of marriage; and we have had financial problems for most of our marriage. And given all this, it is no surprise that my wife and I have experienced marriage trouble.

> "And most of all we are close—probably as close as any family I know. Maybe the trials brought us together."

But even with all these problems, we have experienced a lot of joy and laughter in our family. And most of all we are close—probably as close as any family I know. Maybe the trials brought us together. One thing I know for sure is that my family is my greatest source of joy. I continually thank God for them—they mean everything to me.

For some strange reason I thought my children were off limits in terms of tragedies. I'm not sure why. Of course, I knew in my mind that life is uncertain, and that no one knows the number of their days. But for some reason I thought that when it came to *my* family it was different. Maybe I just didn't want to think about the possibilities, or maybe it was because I was secretly keeping a balance sheet with God. "Okay God, we suffered this, this, and this...so I know You would never let anything happen to my children, right?"

Wrong! On the night of November 4, 2005, the line was crossed. My bubble burst. My house of cards crumbled. It was a Friday night so the children were staying up late. I had gone to bed. My youngest daughter, Emily, had a friend over and they were playing around. My 11-year-old son, Joshua, was joining in the fun. Suddenly my son collapsed on my wife, Becky. She thought he was just being silly, but she quickly realized something was terribly wrong. He was trying to tell her something, but his words were slurred. He seemed to be losing consciousness. In a state of panic, my wife woke me up. I held my son and asked him to tell me what was wrong. He was barely conscious at this point; he kept lifting his hand to his head. He was also convulsing like he was going to vomit. I asked him to tell me how he felt. His last words to me before becoming unconscious were, "I feel sad."

My wife immediately called for an ambulance. Although they arrived quickly, they had difficulty stabilizing him. Finally, after what seemed like an eternity, the ambulance sped away with my wife and son. I followed behind in our van, scared of what I would face when I arrived at the hospital.

I knew immediately that it was serious. Every other time that I had gone to the emergency room it turned into a waiting game. Only real "emergencies" are whisked back for immediate attention. They had already taken my son back and were doing whatever doctors do with such cases. In shock and scared, my wife and I were taken to a private waiting room, not having a clue what was wrong with our son.

I don't know how long we waited. Time seemed to stop. It was like a dream, a very bad dream. Finally, the doctors called us into the room where our son lay unconscious and motionless. A boy who only a couple of hours before had been so full of life—a boy who, in fact, rarely stopped moving or making noise!

As they informed us of what had happened to our son, my heart sank into my stomach. My whole world caved in. Josh had suffered a *severe* brain hemorrhage. Unknown to us, he had been born with a congenital brain defect called an artereovenous malformation (AVM). Although the defect itself is not extremely uncommon—anyone could have one and not know it—only 2-4% of those with the defect result in spontaneous hemorrhages like our son's.

The doctors told us that he was bleeding in his brain and that the pressure had caused him to collapse and become unconscious. His only hope was an emergency brain surgery to stop the bleeding and remove the AVM. My wife and I listened and we understood, but we couldn't believe what we were hearing. Brain surgery! This was something that you watch on TV, or read about in Readers Digest. This wasn't *our* life, and *our* son that this was happening to.

After a sleepless night in the hospital waiting room, the neurosurgeon finally came to us. He cautiously told us that the surgery went well, and that he had done everything he could do. However, he seemed careful not to say anything to get our hopes up. I regretted the few questions that we did ask about his prognosis. In fact, the surgeon left us very discouraged and uncertain about whether or not our son would live at all, let alone be "normal." We were bombarded with thoughts like: Is he going to live? If he does live will he be normal? Will the Josh we know and love return, and if so, when?

I really don't know why we, or any other Christian in such a situation, ask such questions. I suppose one asks hoping to hear good news, or maybe it's just that we would rather "know," however terrible it may be, than live with the uncertainty. However, I've come to learn through this experience that there are as many opinions as there are doctors and that it is better to not ask. Besides, as Christians, our hope should be in God and not humans. Does it really matter what the doctors say? They are, after all, only human.

Believe me; I'm not questioning the value of human medicine. By the grace of God and their expertise my son is still with us today. My point is that doctors are like everyone else; they have their own perspective on a particular situation. While some may see the glass half full, others may see the glass half empty.

Struggling to Maintain Hope...

When I walked into the room to see my son after the surgery, I couldn't believe my eyes. The son that I had watched enter the world—had taught to ride a bike and skateboard, had played football and soccer with, and had watched grow into a normal, healthy, sometimes wild boy—laid lifeless before me. His head was bandaged and swollen, and a myriad of machines with tubes ran into his mouth and veins. It was the saddest day of my life. I sat down and put my head between my legs to keep from fainting. Words cannot describe what I felt at that moment.

What followed was a haze of ups and downs, hopes and let-downs. The doctor's primary concern was the swelling in his brain. If the pressure increased too much it would cut off the oxygen supply to the brain, resulting in permanent damage and possibly death. There was also the risk of a stroke following the surgery. Josh seemed stable the first day after the surgery but our hopes were quickly dashed. My wife called early the second day to tell me that Josh had suffered a stroke during the night which caused the pressure in his cranium to increase.

The neurosurgeon inserted a "bolt" in Josh's head to drain the excess fluid, and to monitor the inter-cranial pressure (ICP). The doctors and nurses battled the pressure for several more days, trying everything possible including lowering his body temperature and putting him into an artificial coma. But by the fourth day it became clear that nothing was working. The ICP remained too high despite all their efforts. The doctors decided that another surgery was necessary. They informed us that the surgeon was going to perform a procedure where part of the brain would be removed and a hole would be left in the cranium to alleviate the pressure. Although the doctors tried to reassure us by telling us that anyone could lose part of their frontal lobe and be "normal," I was not convinced. How could someone lose a sizable portion of their brain and still be okay?

This was my lowest point. My hope had fluctuated but I had never truly despaired. What the doctors were suggesting seemed like desperate measures to me. I honestly believed that my son was going home to be with the Lord. I took a walk and gave him to God (again), thinking that this was really the end. The depth of my grief at that point was inexpressible.

The surgeon that performed the first surgery did this one as well. For some reason, he seemed relatively positive about the results, at least more so than the first surgery. By this time, however, we were already growing skeptical of the doctors' opinions. We had also learned to not ask too many questions.

For the next week we watched the ICP and prayed unceasingly. Finally, the pressure began to stabilize and then gradually decrease. Although the doctors spoke of progress, his condition looked the same from my perspective. He still lay there unconscious and motionless after two weeks. They removed the bolt from Josh's head, which seemed like a positive step, but then they talked to us about installing a tracheotomy and a feeding tube. Again, the doctors tried to reassure us, but deep down I really believed that they were doing this because they didn't think my son would get better—that he would remain in this lifeless, vegetative state. I thought to myself, "Why else would someone need to have a tracheotomy and feeding tube?"

Slowly, Josh's condition improved over the next week or so, to the point where he could leave the ICU and begin rehabilitation. After two and half weeks in the pediatric intensive care unit, my wife and son headed off to Atlanta to begin the long road of rehabilitation. This sounded like good news. Surely they must believe that recovery was possible, or they wouldn't send him to rehab. But when I looked at my son I couldn't see what therapists could possibly do for him. He wasn't even conscious; how could they possibly "work" with him?

Rehab?

The first time I came to visit my son in rehab my heart sank into my stomach again. It was almost as bad as the first time I saw him after his surgery. He was slumped over in a wheelchair, lifeless and drooling. It was like my faith had crashed into a mountain. By all appearances, recovery, even minimal, seemed remote. Sure, some of the doctors and nurses tried to comfort us with stories of other children who had recovered from similar injuries. Of course we desperately wanted to believe that our son would someday become one of the success "stories." But in the back of my mind there were still haunting questions: Did that child have a stroke? Did they remove part of the brain? How high was the ICP, and for how long? How could he possibly recover from this state? Josh seemed far beyond human medicine to me. I thought to myself, "If my son is going to get better, then God, You are the one who's going to have to do it."

For the first time in my life, I literally had no choice but to trust God. I realized that up to this point I had only "played at" trusting in God, but all the while I was trusting in myself. Sure, many times my back had been against the wall, but I always plotted a way out if God didn't come through. This way of coping had been ingrained in me since childhood. My parents who were not Christians had a fairly "hands off" approach to raising children. And since they had separated when I was eight, I had pretty much been left to take care of my-

> "I realized that up to this point I had only "played at" trusting in God, but all the while I was trusting in myself."

self. It wasn't that my parents didn't love me (although I wasn't sure at the time); it was just that they believed that love entailed freedom.

Having independence so deeply ingrained in me, I had struggled with trusting in God since becoming a Christian. Despite the hardships, I continued to believe in and seek God as best I could, but God knew (and I knew as well) that deep down I was holding back. Now for the first time with my son in what seemed like an impossible situation, I was forced to either act on my faith and trust God or give in to despair. The day after it happened I wrote in my journal:

> Now I have the opportunity to put into action
> what I claim to believe. No matter what, God is good
> and He sits on the throne, high above all that we can think,
> imagine, or do. Circumstances do not change who
> He is—Praise God! I would not want a God that was blown
> around by circumstances like me. My son lies in critical
> condition at this moment—He is yours. Thy will be done!
> Only give me the grace and strength to endure your will.[2]

Don't misunderstand me; I'm not suggesting that God did this to my son to make a point, only that this is what God revealed to me through this tragedy. I felt like I was "hanging in the balance of the reality of time," as Bob Dylan sang.[3] There was only today, only this moment. If I look back and think about how my son used to be, I despair. If I look to the future in expectation, I am faced with the demon of uncertainty. So I sat desperately clinging to God to carry me through each moment of every day.

Although it is a constant struggle to keep "casting my burdens on the Lord" (Psalm 55:22), I am beginning to realize the freedom of doing so. For once in my life, there is absolutely nothing I can do. This knowledge is both the source of my suffering—because I want so desperately to do something to help my son —and the source of my liberation. That is, I realize that there really is nothing

I can do but trust in God. The burden is on Him and not me. All I can do is to choose to trust Him, or not.

I think that ultimately this is why what happened to my son has been so devastating. Of course, any parent would be shaken and upset to see their child like this. However, the depth of my suffering transcends this fact. Moreover, I have my wife to compare myself to. She responded entirely differently to what happened to our son. For the most part she simply accepted the circumstances and did whatever was necessary to help him get better. Overall, my wife was a pillar of strength for the first six months.

Maybe this is "normal" for the mothering instinct to take over in such circumstances, and for the father to feel helpless. I obviously have no other experience to compare this to. I suppose that ultimately it doesn't matter any-way; I still have to come to grips with the situation regardless of what others have experienced.

One thing that has become painfully clear through this ordeal is that my faith was not grounded in God. If it had been, I would not feel so empty and lost. Regardless, because my trust was in something else (namely myself), I fell hard and I am still falling. I have not, however, given up. If I had, I wouldn't even bother writing. I am hoping and praying that I recover the true source of my faith—my Lord and Savior, Jesus Christ. Right now I cannot see, or even imagine the end because the darkness is so thick. Nevertheless, I hope and be-lieve that my God will "catch me" and that I will one day walk in the light (with my son) again.

I write in part as an attempt to find that light—the light of my Savior. As an introspective person, I tend to internalize things and mull them over (and over, and over) until I can make sense of them. That, however, is the problem with this situation. The more I try to make sense of it, the less it makes sense. I don't know if it's even possible, yet I don't know how else to cope. Sure, I've given it to God—it seems like a thousand times since it happened—but to no avail in terms of obtaining the relief that I so disparately seek. The gnawing feeling in my stomach remains and the cloud of uncertainty continues to hover over my head. I can see no light.

Reflections

I became pretty depressed at the slow progress that Josh was making along with the separation from Becky and the responsibility of taking care of our daughters (which I was failing at). My biggest frustration, however, was that I could not *do* anything to fix this situation. Becky was the one helping Josh with the things he needed, but I wasn't doing anything. I felt like a useless appendage, which only made things worse.

> "My biggest frustration, however, was that I could not do anything to fix this situation."

Finally, things got so bad that I went to our family doctor for my depression and inability to sleep. This was a big mistake; in hindsight I should have gone to a psychiatrist for this medication. I was taking drugs for my other health problems, and I needed the expertise of a specialist to guide me to the right medications, and dosages.

I don't know if what we experienced, in terms of having a child traumatically injured, was typical but I would think so. I think Becky went into "mother-mode" when Josh was injured and stayed busy taking care of him, while I was stuck on the sidelines watching, unable to do anything to help. Looking back, I see how much Becky needed me and how I could (and should) have supported her, but at the time I was completely blinded by grief. Thankfully, when Becky had her meltdown in May of 2006, I was able to help out more. It finally looked like Josh was going to be "okay" and I felt a lot better about the situation. I was thankful to have our son with us again. However, Becky's grief was just beginning.

Becky

I had many of the same gut-wrenching feelings that Tyler was going through early on. I just kind of survived the first few weeks but was encouraged when Josh was able to speak about six weeks after the hemorrhage. However, I seemed to go into a form of autopilot when things became a little more routine. When Josh was moved to rehab, I remember thinking, "Why am I not falling apart?" I felt semi-detached from all the turmoil and able to do the things I needed to do to help Josh.

I lived at Ronald McDonald House for months starting in the third week. Every day (and night) was consumed with helping Josh get better. I encouraged him as much as I could to keep working and doing what the doctors and specialists asked him to do. We were able to bring Josh home on March 16, 2006, which was about 19 weeks after the crisis.

Tyler did not handle this crisis well. Each time he visited us at the hospital or at the rehabilitation clinic he fell apart. He couldn't even be around Josh without crying. While I was with Josh in Atlanta, Tyler was at home with the girls, but they were pretty much on their own. Tyler slipped into a state of depression. He went to our family doctor who prescribed medication to help him sleep and to help with his depression. The dosage, however, was not right and it turned Tyler into a "zombie." Tyler was even less help, which increased my frustration.

I wanted to talk to Tyler about what was going on with Josh and with our daughters, but he just could not handle it. I felt completely alone during this time. Yes, friends attempted to comfort me but I knew they couldn't understand how I felt. The one person that I knew could understand was my husband but we simply couldn't communicate because he was so devastated. By May of 2006, I was emotionally and physically exhausted. I crashed. I was grief stricken and depressed. Fortunately, Tyler was able to step in at this point and take over managing the family and helping Josh.

One of the strangest outcomes of this crisis is that I have lost much of my sense of empathy for the problems of others. Nor am I as open with others as I was before the crisis. I hold back my feelings in relationships and consequently have difficulty making friends which had always been easy for me. Part of the problem is that I simply don't have time for friends. My days (and many nights) are still centered around Josh's therapy or school. But also, I have this feeling of not wanting to be dependent on others like I have been in the past. I know that I used to lean on other people too much and now I'm trying to lean on God—to trust Him and take my burdens to Him. I think I have learned a few things about dependence on

> "I know that I used to lean on other people too much and now I'm trying to lean on God—to trust Him and take my burdens to Him."

God. I had no choice really; there was no one else. I realize, just as Tyler has, that I am not really in control. This can be both liberating and scary, depending on the day. I remember turning to God at one point in the crisis and saying, "God, if You want Josh, I am willing to give him up to You." But honestly I don't know if I really meant it. I don't know if I could have handled losing my son.

I did ask God if he would keep Josh as he is now. I felt like I lost my little boy forever. He went into a coma and came out very different. Josh went through puberty as he was recovering from his hemorrhage, and I think this complicated his rehab and certainly added to the emotional strain on him and myself. Of course I love him and I'm thankful that he is with us, but I still grieve over the loss of my little boy. It's like he grew up over night.

Josh has continued to improve to the point where he can walk fairly well, although he wears a brace on his ankle because he can't lift his left foot up. He has worked hard in therapy but still has no use of his left arm or hand. His speech, however, is normal except when he talks too fast or is tired. The injury set him back significantly in school, but the public school system has been very accommodating and helpful. He currently receives homebound teaching and is doing well.

Although Josh appears to be a normal 15-year-old, laughing and having fun, he has trouble understanding subtle inferences and jokes. He takes things very literally most of the time, and this can lead to some communication problems, especially with sarcasm. We have to remind him that the person is joking.

The best support, outside the family, that we have is our local church. Josh is active in the youth group and was able to participate at a junior high sleep over camp last summer. He's been talking about next year's camp ever since it ended! He also goes to the weekly youth group meetings and to Sunday school at the church. His sisters have continued to be accepting and supportive of their brother. However, they have each dealt with it in their own way. I think we are only now seeing how much effect this has had on our family as a whole. Our daughters essentially lost their parents for a year or so.

One of the most difficult things for us to consider is Josh's future. Of course, we are hopeful; he is still developing and progressing in school and therapy. The truth is, only God knows. But regardless, it's clear that Josh will most likely have some limitations. Our hope and prayer is that he will be able to live an independent life, make a living, and have a family like he wants to do.

There are many little frustrations that have to be dealt with. For example, Josh wanted to wear flip flops like other teenagers, but they kept falling off. We were able to find a set of sandals that looked similar, but would not fall off. This really made Josh happy, feeling like he was like everyone else.

Tyler spends most of his free time with Josh now—hiking, camping, going to movies, eating out, etc. They have become good friends. While Tyler still grieves about what happened, he is grateful that Josh survived his ordeal and is able to be with the family. There is still much physical and emotional healing that needs to take place. We are confident that Josh will continue to grow and heal as will each of us and our family as a whole.

Four Years Later...

It's been four years since Josh's injury. In many ways the incident itself seems surreal—like a bad dream. The shock and trauma of what happened has largely dissipated. Although we still have moments when we get upset, we have, for the most part, accepted the situation and are doing our best to move on.

Josh has made tremendous progress both mentally and physically. Given the extent of his injury, he truly is a miracle. Statistically, over 95 percent of people who enter the hospital with his symptoms end up either dead or incapacitated for life. When I (Tyler) am tempted to look at Josh's deficiencies, I remind myself of this fact.

Josh continues weekly sessions of physical, occupational, and speech therapy. He walks with an ankle brace (AFO) because he has the "foot-drop" typical of stroke patients. His major physical impairment is the paralysis in his left arm and hand. Although progress in this area seemed to plateau after a year or so, I continued to research and seek out new therapies for his arm and hand.

After trying a number of different orthotic devices and therapies, we seem to have finally found something that is helping—a functional electrical stimulation device, which has led to more progress in one month than in the last three years. This is truly a breakthrough and gives us hope for Josh's continued recovery.

Josh has homebound school offered through the public school district. We had many concerns about Josh attending a large high school, so this is a real blessing. All of the teachers come to our house for his classes. Although Josh is considerably behind grade wise, he continues to make progress.

We are protective of Josh, but we by no means keep him in a box. He's very involved with our church's youth group where he feels completely accepted. He also enjoys many activities, such as playing Frisbee golf and basketball, and hiking and camping. To most people Josh seems like a regular high school teenager with his "cool" clothes and shoes.

Along with being a typical wife and mother (our youngest daughter is still at home), Becky remains busy taking Josh back and forth to therapy, doing his home therapy exercises with him, and coordinating school. She is largely responsible for Josh's progress as she continues to encourage and help him when he is tempted to give up. This has been an ongoing struggle for her to keep Josh motivated as he understandably often grows weary after four years of rigorous therapy.

We are both concerned about Josh's future—how far will he progress? Will he be able to go to college? To live independently? To marry and have a family? For the most part, we just try not to think about it and to focus on the day. We are encouraged because Josh continues to make progress, and the truth is no one knows how much he will recover. This is a concern for Josh as well, and he speaks about it often. We do our best to encourage him and tell him that we believe that God has a plan for his life, emphasizing the importance of developing a relationship with Him.

Chapter Take-a-ways:

Surrender your child and the situation to God.

Be there for each other as a family and talk about your feelings.

Learn to handle frustration with not being able to "fix it."

Discover the importance of maintaining hope.

References:

1 Journal entry November 8, 2005.

2 Journal entry November 5, 2005.

3 "Every Grain of Sand"

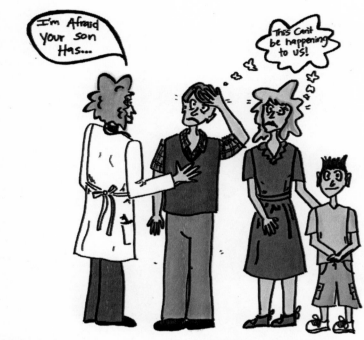

CHAPTER 14

What Is Success?

183

I have struggled with this question for decades. As a young, single person, my idea of success was a great job, a romantic wife, and lots of money for cars, to travel, and buy a nice house. As the realities of life had their impact, I have moved towards more modest financial goals and a very different set of personal goals centered around growth and serving others. Each of us has a different concept of success. This concept drives our behaviors perhaps more than all other things. If we want to be important, we seek a position of authority; if we want to be wealthy, we seek ways to gather money. If we want power, we seek ways to influence people; and if we want to serve others, we seek ways to be supportive and to build others up. Others just want to be content or happy and may do things to avoid conflicts and challenges. Some just seek acceptance or love. Still others seek pleasure in eating, sexual experiences, drugs, alcohol, etc., and will feel successful when they are doing these things.

It Starts in the Mind

Plato said many centuries ago that a life unexamined is worthless. As we look at our life with a child with special needs, the situation screams at us to figure out how we can be successful in this situation. Most of us never contemplated having a child with a disability and so we did not prepare ourselves. It is a shock and forces us to think about the consequences and its impact on our desire to be successful.

Perhaps the most important thought we have about success is the desire to be significant, to do something with our life that is important, long lasting, and worthwhile. Significance can be defined as our being a powerful influence in society or it can be gaining wealth with all the material possessions that impress others. It can be celebrity status as an actor or politician. Significance can also be defined by how many people's lives you make a difference in. Most of us will not be rich, powerful, or be a celebrity, but we can be significant by making a difference in the lives of others. The most important people in your life are your family, your friends, and your co-workers. In your special situation the family includes making the child with special needs a priority while balancing your relationship with your spouse and other children. Any discussion of significance has to include the questions of: Who am I and why do I exist?

What is one of the first things you ask a person you have just met? For many, it is what they do for a living. They respond by telling you their occupation and immediately follow with asking you the same question. Frequently we define ourselves by the way we provide for our family. It is the thing we spend the most time in our week doing. Unfortunately, with the dynamics of the marketplace many parents have had to face the loss of a job and frequently more than once. If your job defines your identity, then you are allowing others to define you, and they can decide to take that away at any time.

In my personal life, I have had many different full-time jobs and three major career changes. I have been an Air Force officer, an engineer, a consultant, a purchasing manager, a general manager, and a university professor. However, my job is *not* who I am. I am a husband, a father, a son, a teacher, and a believer. I am a supporter of others, a provider, and a spiritual person.

Does this in any way answer the question of why I exist? The answer is a resounding no! If you really think about it, you have to exist for a reason. Look at all your skills and abilities. Do they exist just so you can work and raise a family, enjoy life for a while, and then be gone? Most Americans believe in a life after death. Could it be that this life is just a training ground for the next life? If so, are your skills and talents something to be developed and sharpened, or are they gifts that are thrown away at death?

What Is Success?

Perhaps a great way to look at your idea of success is to imagine you are at a funeral—*your* funeral. What are people saying about you? You are gone from this world. Does it matter how many expensive toys you owned, the car you drove, or the house you lived in? Does it matter what jobs you had or how much pleasure you had in your life? As the old saying goes, "You cannot take it with you." What is your legacy? Your legacy is what impact you had on others. They are still around, but you are not. They will judge you by who you were, not by what you had. What greater legacy is there than to have given your life to helping others? Some of the most admired people in modern times are those that served others like Gandhi, Billy Graham, and Mother Teresa.

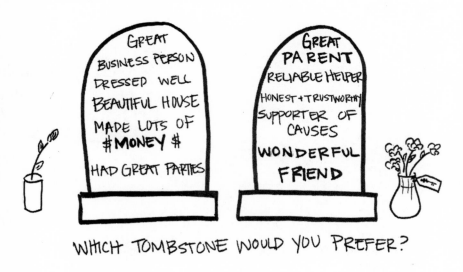

WHICH TOMBSTONE WOULD YOU PREFER?

When we die, we will likely get a tombstone over our grave picked out by our family. Given a choice, which tombstone do you want to have over your grave? The choice is yours to make right now. You decide by what you focus your resources, abilities, talents, and energy on doing for the rest of your life.

Another way to look at success is by what you have accomplished. Worthy accomplishments may include a prestigious job or being responsible for building a bridge or a company, owning a great house and expensive cars and, for a very few of us, coming up with something new. Some of these accomplishments may easily outlast you. The only truly long-lasting impact you are likely to have is on people. Real success may be what you have done to make those who *follow after you* successful. This way you can have an impact over many generations.

Perhaps one of the saddest types of success is the person who does something really well—but it is the wrong type of success. Clearly people who cheat in the stock market, manipulate other people, steal, or kill can fall into this group.

> "Real success may be what you have done to make those who *follow after you* successful."

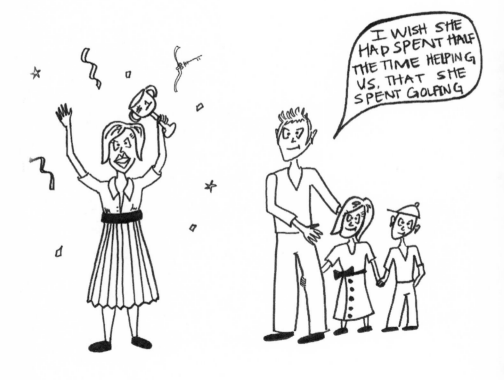

But what about us? Some people seem to be naturally competitive. They focus their time and talent and energy on competing with others. Many companies encourage competition among their workers (car dealerships come to mind). It is not bad to be a successful salesman or trucker, but so often it becomes the primary focus. For the parents of a child with special needs, an over focus on competitive activities can tend to leave the family as a secondary interest.

How common is it for a man to be successful in the marketplace but completely fail as a father and as a husband? How common is it for a woman to be great at her job or have a great social life but fail as a mother or a wife? How many great amateur golfers (or any other type of recreation or sport) are out there that focus all their energies on the sport instead of where it really matters? The scratch golfer will be easily forgotten in a few weeks and the 220 level bowler likewise. The conqueror of a role-playing video game will be forgotten as soon as the next version comes out. Great parties will be forgotten in days. However, the parent who helps others be successful may leave a true legacy. We urge you to use your skills for what really matters. Just because you have great talent at playing cards or swimming or running does not mean you have to use that skill to the fullest or even a lot. You have many other skills to use also. These skills may not be as outstanding as some others you have, but they may be more important to use.

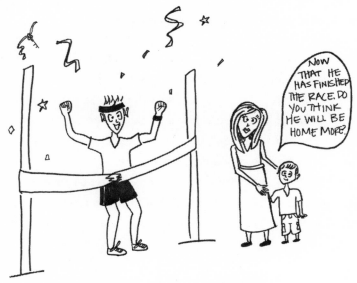

You have a child with a disability. You have many talents, skills, and abilities that can make a huge difference in your child's life. Can you contemplate what that success might be, using those skills and abilities for the purpose of helping your family and your children? Maybe the special child in your life is there to challenge you and to help you focus your efforts in sharpening your skills – skills that can be long lasting and maybe even have eternal benefits.

Virtually none of us would have chosen for our son or daughter to be disabled or to become disabled. It is, however, the way it is. In most cases, you cannot change this situation; you just have to deal with it. The testing and the challenges can and will lead to perseverance and added strength. In Hebrews 10:36 (NIV) we read, "You need to persevere so that when you have done the will of God, you will receive what he has promised." We are better parents, spouses, teachers, and leaders now because of the challenge of raising Brent. You can have great skills, but if you do not use them and sharpen them, they waste away. In this sense, your child with special needs is a blessing to you. You can return that blessing by being the best parent you can be.

> "You can have great skills, but if you do not use them and sharpen them, they waste away. In this sense, your child with special needs is a blessing to you."

But what about those of us who think we have few skills and abilities? It is hard to sharpen something that does not exist, right? However, the good news is that each of us can develop our character. We can become more patient, kinder, gentler, more supportive, more peaceful, and exhibit greater self-control. You can be a great parent just by hanging in there and doing what you can to help. You do not have to be a world renowned expert in the disability or a great physical therapist to help your child. Just doing your part can make a huge difference. Be a good provider, maintain the home, give your spouse a break from the grind, help with the other children, etc. Do what you can and do it to the best of your abilities. This is what is truly impressive. Doing the best with what you have is perhaps the greatest achievement anyone can ever attain!

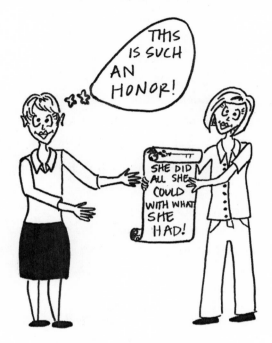

Troubled Times

Most of us can cope in our lives during times of relative stability. However, what about those times when everything is falling apart, and all at the same time? This is when we hope to have reserve energy, people to help us, extra money in the bank to use, etc. Perhaps the greatest thing we really need in times of trouble is *strength of character*. Who does not admire the person who never seems to be shaken no matter the circumstances? Who does not admire people who do their best, and give it their best shot? A key question is, where does this strength of character come from?

The good news is that each of us can develop strength of character. Character is developed over time; it is not generally developed during a crisis. A crisis may reveal a person's true character as it so often does, but character is not usually *created* by the crisis. Development comes from the many small things we deal with in life. How we handle a crying child, a temporary money shortage, a sick relative, forced overtime at work, etc., will develop our character. These routine situations will happen many times and give you many chances to improve how you respond to them. Over 2,700 years ago, the prophet Isaiah wrote: "It seems it was good for me to go through all those troubles," (Isaiah 38:17, The Message). If you mess up, as we all do, you are likely to get a second, a third, and a fourth chance to do better. Doing better each time is developing your character.

The single parent is certainly forced to develop character perhaps faster than anyone else in this situation. Typically there are fewer resources, less time, and no one to share the burdens with. The challenges are yours and yours alone. Thankfully, most of the single parents we know have been able to get through even very difficult times. They have developed the fortitude and the character to handle all that has been thrown their way. Most are better and stronger people for the experiences.

The development of character will then help you to handle the dying parent, the layoff from your job, the visit to the emergency room, and the wrecked car. The routine challenges we face develop our ability to handle the inevitable crises that we will all face in our lifetimes. If the crisis occurs before we have had a chance to develop

> "Even though the crisis of a disability is significant, *it will probably not be the greatest crisis you will face. What you learn from this experience can be great preparation for the future.*"

a strong character, then we can be devastated by it. This is what happens to so many parents when they face the sudden crisis of learning that their child has a disability. As was discussed earlier, this is not the time to give up. It is a time of forced growth. Even though the crisis of a disability is significant, *it will probably not be the greatest crisis you will face.* What you learn from this experience can be great preparation for the future.

Thoughts on Success

Another way of looking at success is in terms of just doing what is right. If each of us always did what we knew was right all the time, it would be hard to argue that we were not being successful. However, in many situations, we can have difficulty knowing the right thing to do. For instance, should a manager fire a problem employee who seems to be trying hard? (Many of our children with disabilities will create situations like this for *their* employers). Do we, as a sales person, take an order we are not sure the company can deliver on the promise date? Should we go over the head of our son's teacher to get what we want, but with the likely result of antagonizing her?

There is a rule that can help us make good decisions. The rule is to do unto others as you would have them do unto you. If you were the employee, would you want to be fired? If you were the customer, would you want to place the order if it will not be delivered on time? If you were the teacher, would you want to have parents making you look bad to your principal? By placing yourself in the other person's position, you can frequently know what the right decision is. Good decision making is a way to become a successful person.

Another point to make here is that you are a role model for your children, for your family, and for almost everyone you come in contact with. Others are watching you make those right decisions. Research shows that children learn values and morals not from what they are taught, but from what they observe others *doing.* The same principle applies in the workplace as employees watch what executives do, not what they say. It is impossible to teach honesty if you make false claims on your tax return. Integrity is impossible to pass on to another person if you do not act in an ethical way in your dealings with them. Ethics, morals,

> "We are willing to bet that the most admired people in your life are the ones that act with integrity and are willing to do the right thing in all types of situations."

and values are "caught," not "taught." Think of the persons you most admire. We are willing to bet that the most admired people in your life are the ones that act with integrity and are willing to do the right thing in all types of situations. They treat others as they would like to be treated themselves. You can trust them and you feel good dealing with them. Why not be like them? You can "catch" their success.

Trust

Trust is a key issue for your family. To be a successful parent, it is critical to be trusted by your spouse, your children, and your extended family. Trust is especially important to your child with a disability as he or she is so dependent on you. If the child cannot trust you, it puts him or her in a very difficult situation. One of the things that all children crave is security, knowing they are safe and knowing that the adults in their lives are going to be there when they need them. To feel secure, a child, especially a child with disabilities, needs to be able to trust you absolutely. They need to know that your word is always true, that you will not fail them when they need you, and that you will do whatever you can to help them.

Trust is earned by the day-to-day way you live and interact with your family. It does not take many untrustworthy acts to ruin that trust. In addition, if trust is lost, then the child will lose his or her sense of security. Loss of trust and security can lead to tremendous psychological problems. The child with a disability probably already feels less secure than most other children. To be a successful parent, you must do your absolute best to be there when they need you, to be reliable, and to do the right thing in all circumstances. Do for them what you would want someone to do for you.

We believe that almost all parents want to do what is best for their children. However, many are not successful because of the influences of friends and advisors. Good character can be negatively influenced by the presence of unethical, mean, or self-absorbed people. Executives cook the books because their associates say they can get away with it. Coworkers encourage people to go to their favorite "watering holes" after work, and singles encourage married people to act more like them. The world is full of people that are going to encourage you to make other things a higher priority than your family. If you choose to spend time with people that are not of high integrity and strong character, then you risk being dragged down to their level. As the old saying goes, "You cannot soar like an eagle when you run with the turkeys."

> "If you choose to spend time with people that are not of high integrity and strong character, then you risk being dragged down to their level."

What you learn from your life experiences can also be great preparation for eternity. The most popular Christian book of recent times is *The Purpose Driven Life* by Rick Warren. Reportedly, there have been over 30 million copies of this book sold. In the book, Warren discusses the reasons we exist and how to become the person God designed you to be. One of his key points is that we were shaped for service and we need to develop our many talents to serve others and to serve God. He points out early in the book that our life on earth is a temporary assignment. During this temporary assignment, we are supposed to develop our character. It may be hard to accept, but the difficulties we face today may be a blessing to us if we can be strengthened by them! I highly recommend this book if you are unsure of why you are here and why you are dealing with the problems you have. I read the book once on my own and again as I led a study of the book with my men's group.

A Final Thought

One of the greatest Christian leaders of the 20th century was Norman Vincent Peale. He wrote many books, with the most famous being *The Power of Positive Thinking*. One of his critical concepts was that the secret of life is not in what actually happens to you, but is more what you do with what happens to you. We are each given a different set of circumstances and challenges to face in our life. Success may not be in the observable results that occur in our lifetime. Rather it may be more about how we deal with those circumstances and challenges. Success may be more the process of growing than the actual outcome.

We can all look at things in our life and say this or that was not fair. Having a child with a disability is certainly not fair, at least in comparison to families with apparently normal children. However, just suppose that you were given this challenge just so you could learn from it, grow from it, and develop your character from it. Success would be measured, not in how well the children in the family did, but rather in how you did. Whom did this experience turn you into? What abilities and talents were developed? How much better is your character because of this experience?

If you choose not to face this situation, you may never know the person you could have been. Failure happens to all of us. However, the key is not the failure – it is what we learn from the failure. This is great wisdom. True success may be measured in each of us by what wisdom we have learned and what this wisdom has done to change us.

Chapter Take-a-ways:

Be trustworthy.

Do the things you know are right.

Develop the strength of your character.

What do you want your tombstone to say?

References

Peale, N. (1978). *The power of positive thinking*. Pawling, NY: Peale Center for Christian Living.

Warren, R. (2002). *The purpose driven life*. Grand Rapids, MN: Zonderman.

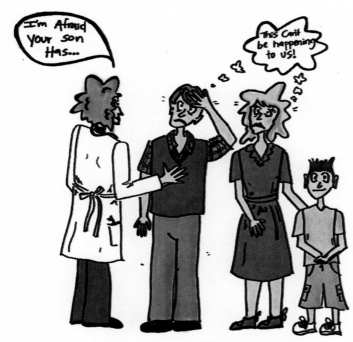

CHAPTER 15
RATE, Vision, & Peace

199

Each of us is provided four things to use in life. I have put these into the acronym of RATE. Each of us is given a set of **R**esources, a set of **A**bilities, a certain amount of **T**ime, and a limited amount of **E**nergy to deal with *all* of life's problems. Obviously each of us has a different RATE to work with. Not one of us is the same. Also unique to each of us is our situation. Each of us is in a unique situation, dealing with a unique set of problems, opportunities, and people. So how does anyone get an evaluation of their life in this unique situation? How do we know if we are doing well?

Some parents seem to have a relatively easy life. They have smart children that behave well and do well in school and in sports. They grow up to be good spouses and parents with good jobs and have a number of friends. They are not dealing with the same problems we are dealing with. Perhaps it is because they would not be able to handle the problems we have, or that they could not learn from the experience.

This is playing the comparison game. We already know that everyone is unique and living in a unique situation where comparisons are really meaningless. Everyone has a different RATE. The only way to measure success is in terms of *your* RATE and *your* situation. You can always find another person that seems to win the comparison game, and the comparison is *never* fair. On top of this, the situation and the RATE can change over time. We may start our adult lives with few resources but have a lot of time left in our lives. Later we may have more resources, but less time and energy.

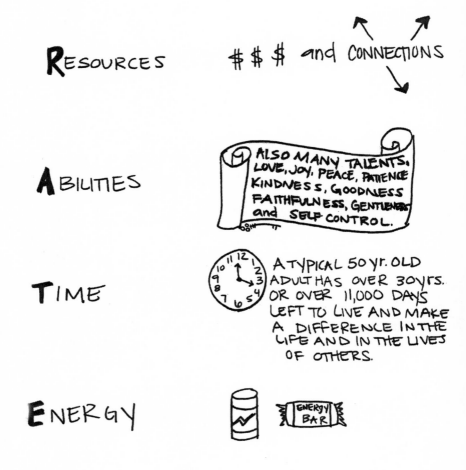

RESOURCES   # $ # and CONNECTIONS

ABILITIES

ALSO MANY TALENTS, LOVE, JOY, PEACE, PATIENCE KINDNESS, GOODNESS FAITHFULNESS, GENTLENESS and SELF CONTROL.

TIME

A TYPICAL 50 yr. OLD ADULT HAS OVER 30 yrs. OR OVER 11,000 DAYS LEFT TO LIVE AND MAKE A DIFFERENCE IN THE LIFE AND IN THE LIVES OF OTHERS.

ENERGY

ENERGY BAR

Your situation involves the raising of a child with special needs. You need to use a lot of your RATE to help the child and the family. You do not have to do so, but I believe most of us know we should. God has given us free will to decide how to use our RATE. It can be used for success in business, sports, or games. You may even earn recognition for your accomplishments in these areas. However, using our RATE only for ourselves is a poor use of these gifts. Not many of us will think a parent successful if he uses his resources, abilities, time, and energy only for himself and neglects his family. The Bible is very clear on this priority. We are to take care of our family (I Timothy 5:8).

The RATE we are given is really a stewardship situation. By this, I mean that the different aspects of our RATE, especially the resources and time, are only temporarily ours. God does not grant anyone unlimited time or resources. When we leave this world our resources go to someone else and by definition we are out of time. We also lose our energy and our abilities as we age. Therefore, we only have our RATE for a limited time. It is a gift to be used for a while, and then it is lost.

Using our RATE to help others is the best way to help ourselves. There is little that feels better than helping others, serving others, and making a positive difference in the lives of others. True success is how well you use your

> "...we only have our RATE for a limited time. It is a gift to be used for a while, and then it is lost."

RATE not just for yourself, but also most importantly for others. When you are in need, don't you want others to help you, to use *their* RATE to help you? Others are looking for help from you right now. Use your RATE to do just that. Your child with a disability certainly needs your RATE in his or her life.

Vision

What is your vision of how you and your family will look next year, in five years, or 20 years? Many of us fail to have a clear vision of what we think will happen. If you do have a vision, it may be pretty cloudy and full of storms. If your child's disability is not curable, or you feel that disability can never be fully compensated for, then this will surely cloud your vision. Everyone has ideas of what the future will look like. If things are not going well, we tend to be either negative or just try not to think about it. This seems to be the most typical situation for many parents. We have a sense of an unknown or an unpleasant future, and we try not to think about it much.

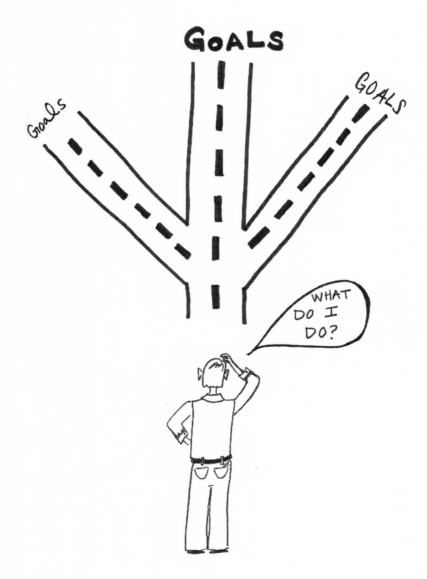

Parents of Children with Disabilities

A vision for the future, of the possibilities of what can happen, is essential to guiding our actions. For the vast majority of us there is a real possibility of a very positive future. Children with even extreme disabilities can still get college degrees and/or hold down good jobs. They can be married and can even have a family. They can become self sufficient and significantly less dependent on you or on the help of others.

Technology in the area of prosthetics (artificial body parts) is advancing rapidly. Artificial vision systems seem to be just around the corner, as does the development of technology such as stem cells to cure many diseases that

> "There seems to be hope in dealing with almost every type of disability."

are beyond our ability to deal with right now. New drugs are being tested for many diseases and new techniques are being developed to deal with so many disabilities. There seems to be hope in dealing with almost every type of disability.

Single parents may not always be single and may have much improved situations in their futures. Just as the child's situation may improve, so may the situation for the parent. Perhaps our country will radically change the current medical health care system, which will change the approach to helping those in need. With prayer and perseverance, anything is possible.

So what is your vision? Developing a vision of what *can be* is essential to guiding your actions now. There is a very old concept that says without vision people will perish (Proverbs 29:18). You must have goals to strive for, or you will never get where you want to be. The old joke goes like this: A driver stops at a gas station and asks for directions. The clerk asks the driver where they are trying to go. The driver responds that they are not sure. Therefore, the clerk tells them it doesn't matter which way they go. Are you like this driver? Are you just taking one day at a time with no real goals in mind? Are you just *hoping* things will somehow get better? If so, then you are not really seeking a winning future for yourself or your family.

Dream or Nightmare?

Put another way, vision without action is just dreaming. However, action without vision can be a nightmare! Sit down with your spouse or significant other, or your friends, and start examining what the future can look like. Plan for success. Set short term goals and longer term goals that can lead to the future you want. Obviously, there will be detours along the way—things that do not go as planned and setbacks. Our long-term goal for our son is for him to be able to live independently, have a regular job, and have a set of friends he can count on. We also want him to be active in his church and to learn relationship skills. We are not there yet. A few years ago, Brent was unsuccessful in his third attempt to live independently. He now has a regular part-time job that has lasted longer than any previous job. Unfortunately, since we moved to Virginia over three years ago, he is not active in a church and is not developing a set of friends. He still has much to learn about relationships. In the fall of 2009 Brent moved into a house by himself. We are seeking at least one other person to live with him to provide some form of friendship.

Life is a journey. To complete your journey you need a destination, but sometimes the vision has to change. Our vision 15 years ago was loftier than it is now. At that time, we hoped Brent could graduate from college, be motivated to hold down a full-time job, and possibly get married. Brent could not pass the English writing exams and so he could not continue in college. He has had several long-term relationships and was even engaged for a brief period of time. Another long-term relationship seems distant at this point. Therefore, we have recast our vision again. We still have a vision and we do all we can to make that vision become reality. Without a clear vision, you cannot be sure that what you are doing is helping or hurting. Again, we believe you need to have a vision for the future and to use that vision to drive your actions now.

Peace

There is nothing more desired by almost everyone I know than peace. We want peace from the tension at work and at home; peace from the people wanting to get something out of us or to sell something to us; peace from all those that want our attention; peace from having to be places we don't really want to be, with people we are not comfortable with; and peace from our family conflicts. We want peace to have time to think and relax without the guilt of knowing we should be doing something else.

Where do you find peace? The ultimate solution is, of course, when our life is over, when we meet our Maker. However, we can also feel at peace when we know we have really tried to use our RATE to bless others. Peaceful people are those that put their self-serving nature behind them and focus on being a blessing to others. Peaceful people put their pride on the shelf and just do the right thing that honors those around them. There is no way to avoid the pressures of life, to rid life of stress. As the parent of a child with special needs you have obligations and numerous demands on your resources, your abilities, your time, and your energy. The real trick is to do what is really important and not to do the things that keep you from doing the important. Put another way, do not let the urgent things in life prevent you from doing the important things in life.

We face a massive demand on our RATE. Many things seem to be urgent and must be dealt with promptly. Our boss asks us to work overtime again. Our friend asks us to do him another favor. The school needs you to help out, and your family forces obligations on you. Maybe you are in debt (the average American family has over $8,000 in credit card debt) and the bills are starting to pile up. All these demands force us to make decisions that are tradeoffs between these urgent things and the things that are really important. *The urgent attempts to overwhelm the important.*

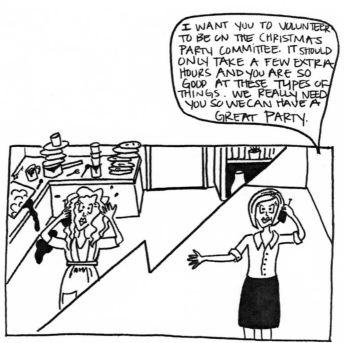

THE URGENT ATTEMPTS TO OVERWHELM THE IMPORTANT

You need to decide what is important and make all your decisions based on those important things. When you start making decisions this way, there is a real sense of peace because you are doing the best you can do and taking care of the important things in life. The world will attempt to flatter you, to insist it needs you for this project or that event. Your "friends" will draw you to spend time with them. The people around you will pressure you to use your RATE for their goals and needs. Guilt will be laid on thickly when you do not do their will. However, if we are taking care of our family, our marriage, and ourselves as important priorities, we can have the peace of knowing that we are doing what is important and right. By making the important decisions now about using your RATE, you have an answer when the world comes knocking.

I do not want to suggest that you use your RATE only for going to work and taking care of your family. The chapters on helping yourself and your marriage clearly point out that you need to have breaks and to have times to relax. Some things the world asks of you are very hard to avoid—especially those related to supporting your family. You may decide it is appropriate to give your RATE to your extended family. The difference is that you know what is really important and you will not compromise the important no matter how urgently the world comes at you. You are at peace because you know what is really important.

True Peace

True peace actually has to come from God. Isaiah 32:17 (NIV) says, "The fruit of righteousness will be peace; the effect of righteousness will be quietness and confidence forever." Righteousness comes only from God—from being right with God. We are Christians, and we find it very difficult to understand how parents who are not Christians cope with the stress. We have the confidence that God cares about us and wants us to be successful in our marriage, with our family and friends, in the work we do, and in helping our son.

The words of Jesus are clear: "I am leaving you with a gift—peace of mind and heart. And the peace I give isn't like the peace the world gives. So don't be troubled or afraid" (John 14:27, NLT). The peace from God is special and cannot be duplicated by anyone or anything. I urge you to give Jesus a chance to bless you and help you. Jesus does *not* promise to free you of your troubles. In John 16:33 (NLT) Jesus says, "I have told you all this so that you may have peace in me. Here on earth you will have many trials and sorrows. But take heart, because I have overcome the world."

Our Lord promises to help us deal with our troubles and to help us grow our character through the experience. His peace is easy to receive if you will acknowledge your need, recognize

> "Our Lord promises to help us deal with our troubles and to help us grow our character through the experience."

His authority over your life, and accept His guidance for your life. The ancient words from 3,000 years ago are still true: "May the Lord bless you and protect you. May the Lord smile on you and be gracious to you. May the Lord show you his favor and give you his peace" (Numbers 6:24-26, NLT).

As a final thought, I urge you again to give Jesus a chance to show you how He can help. This battle is not one you want to fight alone. Get help. The best help in the universe is there for the asking. Do not allow those that profess to be believers, but act just like non-believers, to distract you. Overcome your pride, overcome the hypocrisy, and overcome the doubters. Do it for yourself, for your family, and for your children. Just do it!

Chapter Take-a-ways:

Use your RATE to bless your family.

Develop a vision to guide your actions.

Do not let the urgent overwhelm the important.

Put your trust in the peace Jesus offers you.

CPSIA information can be obtained at www.ICGtesting.com
Printed in the USA
BVOW070707051211

277588BV00001B/4/P